AF354496

Hypertension (High Blood Pressure)

-

From Causes to Control

by

VIRUTI SHIVAN

Masters in Clinical Psychology (Major)

"In books, as in life, it's not the size or looks but the content that matters."

Introduction

Welcome to "Hypertension (High Blood Pressure) - From Causes to Control," a comprehensive guide designed to walk you through every aspect of understanding, managing, and potentially reversing hypertension. This book is more than just a collection of medical advice; it's a journey into the heart of what it means to live with and combat high blood pressure. Through these pages, you'll find a blend of science, personal stories, and practical advice aimed at providing you with the tools you need to take control of your health.

Hypertension is often called the "silent killer" because it can cause significant damage without obvious symptoms. It's a condition that quietly undermines your health, contributing to heart disease, stroke, kidney failure, and other serious problems. Despite its prevalence and severity, many aspects of hypertension remain misunderstood by the general public. That's where this book comes in. We aim to demystify high blood pressure, explaining its causes in understandable terms, outlining the latest treatments, and offering clear strategies for prevention and reversal.

Our journey begins with the basics—what blood pressure is, how it's measured, and what those measurements mean. From there, we delve into the complex web of factors that can lead to hypertension, from genetics to lifestyle choices, and how these elements interact in unique ways for each individual. But understanding the problem is only half the battle; the heart of this book lies in its practical advice for managing and overcoming hypertension.

We'll explore the impact of diet, exercise, and stress management, providing actionable tips and real-life strategies that have proven effective. Medications, their benefits, and potential side effects will be discussed, focusing on generic names to ensure the information remains timeless and universally applicable. We also recognize the power of alternative therapies and the role of personal anecdotes in illustrating the human side of managing hypertension.

By the end of this book, you'll have a thorough understanding of hypertension and a personalized toolkit for addressing it. While we cannot offer illustrations or images due to copyright reasons, we believe the vivid narratives, engaging examples, and clear, concise explanations will paint a picture just as vividly in your mind. This guide is not just about combating a condition; it's about embracing a healthier lifestyle and making informed choices for your future.

As we embark on this journey together, remember that the path to better health is not always linear. There will be challenges and setbacks, but there is also hope and possibility. Whether you're newly diagnosed, a caregiver, or simply interested in maintaining optimal health, this book is for you. Let's begin this journey with an open mind, ready to learn, adapt, and take control of our health, one step at a time.

Chapter 1: Understanding Hypertension

1.1 The Basics of Blood Pressure

Blood pressure is a critical indicator of your overall cardiovascular health, serving as a vital metric that reflects the force of blood pushing against the walls of your arteries. This force is generated with each heartbeat, as blood is pumped from the heart into the arteries to be circulated throughout the body. Understanding the basics of blood pressure is essential for grasping how hypertension develops and why it poses a significant risk to your health.

Blood pressure readings are presented as two numbers: systolic and diastolic. **Systolic blood pressure**, the higher of the two numbers, measures the pressure in your arteries when your heart beats. **Diastolic blood pressure**, the lower number, measures the pressure in your arteries when your heart rests between beats. These measurements are recorded in millimeters of mercury (mmHg) and typically presented as systolic over diastolic (e.g., 120/80 mmHg).

A normal blood pressure reading for most adults is around 120/80 mmHg. Readings above this level may be considered elevated or indicative of hypertension, depending on how much higher they are. The American Heart Association defines hypertension as a consistently high blood pressure reading of 130/80 mmHg or higher.

Several factors can influence your blood pressure, including but not limited to:

- **Age:** Blood pressure typically increases with age due to the hardening of the arteries.

- **Diet:** High sodium intake, low potassium, and excessive alcohol consumption can raise blood pressure.

- **Weight:** Being overweight or obese is a key risk factor for developing hypertension.

- **Activity level:** Lack of physical activity can contribute to higher blood pressure.

- **Stress:** Chronic stress can lead to temporary increases in blood pressure.

Understanding these basics is crucial not only for recognizing the risks associated with high blood pressure but also for appreciating the importance of regular monitoring. By keeping track of your blood pressure, you can identify potential health issues early and take steps to address them. Regular monitoring can also provide valuable feedback on the effectiveness of lifestyle changes or medications intended to lower blood pressure.

In the upcoming sections, we will delve deeper into the causes and risk factors of hypertension, its symptoms and warning signs, and explore exercises designed to test your understanding of this critical health issue. Through a comprehensive approach to understanding blood pressure, you can empower yourself to take proactive steps towards maintaining or achieving optimal cardiovascular health.

1.2 Causes and Risk Factors of Hypertension

Understanding the causes and risk factors of hypertension is key to preventing and managing high blood pressure. Hypertension can arise from a variety of factors, often interplaying in complex ways. Some of these factors are within our control, while others, such as genetics, are not. This section explores the myriad factors contributing to hypertension, offering insight into how they affect blood pressure and what can be done to mitigate their impact.

Genetics: Family history plays a significant role in hypertension. If your parents or other close relatives have high blood pressure, your risk of developing the condition is significantly higher. Although we cannot change our genetic makeup, being aware of our family history can motivate us to adopt healthier lifestyle choices early on.

Age: The risk of hypertension increases with age. As we grow older, our blood vessels naturally begin to stiffen and narrow, which can increase blood pressure. This is why monitoring blood pressure becomes even more crucial as we age.

Diet: A diet high in salt (sodium chloride) can raise blood pressure. Sodium causes the body to retain water, which increases the volume of blood in the bloodstream, leading to higher blood pressure. Conversely, a diet low in potassium can also contribute to hypertension, as potassium helps balance the amount of sodium in your cells.

Obesity and Overweight: Excess body weight forces your heart to work harder to pump blood to the tissues, increasing the pressure on your artery walls. Furthermore, obesity is often associated with other risk factors, such as high cholesterol and insulin resistance, which can further exacerbate hypertension.

Physical Inactivity: A sedentary lifestyle contributes to the development of hypertension by allowing weight gain and reducing the overall efficiency of the heart. Regular physical activity helps lower blood pressure by strengthening the heart, making it more efficient at pumping blood.

Alcohol and Tobacco Use: Excessive alcohol consumption and smoking can raise your blood pressure. Alcohol can temporarily increase blood pressure and also lead to long-term blood pressure issues. Tobacco products contain nicotine, which can narrow your arteries and increase heart rate, raising blood pressure.

Stress: While stress itself may not cause long-term hypertension, it can lead to temporary spikes in blood pressure. Over time, these spikes may cause damage to your blood vessels, heart, and kidneys, contributing to or exacerbating hypertension.

Chronic Conditions: Certain chronic conditions, such as diabetes, kidney disease, and sleep apnea, can increase the risk of developing hypertension. Managing these conditions is crucial for controlling or preventing high blood pressure.

Understanding these causes and risk factors allows individuals to identify areas in their lives that may need adjustment to lower their risk of hypertension. While genetics and age cannot be changed, lifestyle factors such as diet, physical activity, and managing stress can significantly impact blood pressure levels. Awareness and proactive management of these risk factors can lead to better health outcomes and reduce the risk of complications associated with hypertension.

1.3 Symptoms and Early Warning Signs

Hypertension is often termed the "silent killer" because it may not present noticeable symptoms until it has caused significant damage. However, being vigilant about potential symptoms and early warning signs can help in identifying and managing hypertension before it leads to more severe health issues. It's crucial to understand that many people with high blood pressure might not experience any symptoms at all, which is why regular blood pressure checks are important.

Some individuals with elevated blood pressure levels might experience symptoms that could serve as early warning signs, though these are not exclusively indicative of hypertension and can be related to various health conditions. Recognizing these signs can prompt further investigation and early intervention:

- **Headaches:** Frequent, unexplained headaches can sometimes be linked to elevated blood pressure levels, especially if they occur without any apparent cause.

- **Shortness of Breath:** Difficulty breathing or shortness of breath, particularly with exertion or at rest in severe cases, can be associated with high blood pressure.

- **Nosebleeds:** Although nosebleeds can be caused by many factors, sudden, unexplained nosebleeds may occasionally be a sign of hypertension, especially if they are recurrent.

- **Vision Changes:** Hypertension can lead to changes in vision, including blurred or double vision, due to its effect on the blood vessels in the eyes.

- **Chest Pain or Discomfort:** High blood pressure can contribute to heart disease, which may manifest as chest pain or discomfort during physical activity or stress.

- **Dizziness:** While dizziness can be caused by a myriad of health issues, it is sometimes related to changes in blood pressure.

- **Fatigue or Confusion:** High blood pressure can affect your energy levels and cognitive function, leading to feelings of fatigue or moments of confusion.

It's important to note that these symptoms can be mild or attributed to other causes, which is why hypertension can go unnoticed for years. The absence of symptoms does not mean the absence of risk. High blood pressure silently and progressively damages the cardiovascular system, kidneys, and other organs, potentially leading to stroke, heart attack, kidney failure, and other serious health conditions.

Given the potential asymptomatic nature of hypertension, the best early warning system is regular monitoring of your blood pressure. This can be done at home with a blood pressure monitor, at a pharmacy, or by a healthcare professional. If high blood pressure is detected early, lifestyle changes and, if necessary, medication can significantly reduce the risk of developing severe complications. Regular health check-ups and being mindful of your body's signals are key steps in preventing and managing hypertension.

1.4 Exercise: 10 MCQs with Answers at the End

Test your understanding of the concepts covered in the first chapter on understanding hypertension with these multiple-choice questions (MCQs). Answers are provided at the end for self-assessment.

1. What does systolic blood pressure measure?

A. The pressure when the heart is at rest

B. The pressure when the heart beats

C. The volume of blood in the bloodstream

D. The resistance of blood flow in the arteries

2. Which of the following is considered a normal blood pressure reading for most adults?

A. 140/90 mmHg

B. 120/80 mmHg

C. 130/85 mmHg

D. 150/95 mmHg

3. What role does sodium play in blood pressure?

A. It decreases heart rate.

B. It causes the body to retain water, increasing blood volume.

C. It strengthens the heart.

D. It decreases blood volume.

4. Which lifestyle factor is NOT associated with increased blood pressure?

A. High sodium diet

B. Regular physical activity

C. Excessive alcohol consumption

D. Smoking

5. Which condition is a known risk factor for developing hypertension?

A. Insomnia

B. Diabetes

C. Hypothermia

D. Hyperactivity

6. What is the primary effect of nicotine on blood pressure?

A. It immediately lowers blood pressure.

B. It causes long-term decreases in blood pressure.

C. It narrows arteries and increases heart rate.

D. It expands arteries and decreases heart rate.

7. **Chronic stress is known to:**

   A. Have no effect on blood pressure.

   B. Cause temporary increases in blood pressure.

   C. Permanently lower blood pressure.

   D. Increase blood volume.

8. **Which of the following is NOT a symptom of hypertension?**

   A. Frequent, unexplained nosebleeds

   B. Sudden, severe lower back pain

   C. Blurred or double vision

   D. Headaches

9. **Regular monitoring of blood pressure is important because:**

   A. Hypertension always presents with clear symptoms.

   B. It helps in the early detection and management of hypertension.

   C. Blood pressure readings are constant and do not fluctuate.

   D. It can replace medication in most cases.

10. Lifestyle changes recommended for managing hypertension include all EXCEPT:

A. Increasing sodium intake.

B. Engaging in regular physical activity.

C. Limiting alcohol consumption.

D. Following a balanced, low-sodium diet.

Answers:

1. **B. The pressure when the heart beats**

2. **B. 120/80 mmHg**

3. **B. It causes the body to retain water, increasing blood volume.**

4. **B. Regular physical activity**

5. **B. Diabetes**

6. **C. It narrows arteries and increases heart rate.**

7. **B. Cause temporary increases in blood pressure.**

8. **B. Sudden, severe lower back pain**

9. **B. It helps in the early detection and management of hypertension.**

10. **A. Increasing sodium intake.**

Chapter 2: Diagnosing Hypertension

2.1 Tools and Techniques for Measurement

The accurate measurement of blood pressure is a cornerstone in diagnosing hypertension, guiding treatment, and monitoring the effectiveness of interventions. This chapter delves into the various tools and techniques used to measure blood pressure, highlighting their importance in the clinical management of hypertension.

Sphygmomanometer and Stethoscope: The traditional method of measuring blood pressure involves a sphygmomanometer, which may be aneroid or mercury-based, and a stethoscope. The cuff of the sphygmomanometer is wrapped around the upper arm and inflated to temporarily stop blood flow in the artery. As the cuff deflates, the practitioner listens with a stethoscope to detect the sounds of blood flow, known as Korotkoff sounds. The first appearance of these sounds corresponds to systolic pressure, and their disappearance marks the diastolic pressure.

Automated Blood Pressure Monitors: Automated or digital blood pressure monitors are widely used in both clinical settings and at home for their ease of use and convenience. These devices typically use the oscillometric method, which detects the oscillations in the arterial wall caused by blood flow as the cuff deflates. Automated monitors display both systolic and diastolic pressures and often include features such as heart rate measurement. While convenient, it's important to ensure these devices are properly calibrated and validated for accuracy.

Ambulatory Blood Pressure Monitoring (ABPM): ABPM involves wearing a blood pressure cuff for 24 hours to obtain measurements throughout the day and night. This method provides a comprehensive profile of an individual's blood pressure, including variations during sleep, periods of activity, and under normal living conditions. ABPM is particularly useful for diagnosing "white-coat hypertension," where a patient's blood pressure is elevated in a clinical setting but normal at home, and "masked hypertension," where the opposite occurs.

Home Blood Pressure Monitoring: Encouraged by healthcare providers, home monitoring involves patients using automated blood pressure devices to track their readings over time. Home monitoring can help in the early detection of hypertension, assess the effectiveness of treatments, and encourage patient engagement in their own care. It's crucial for patients to receive proper training on technique and device selection to ensure accurate readings.

Regardless of the method used, accurate blood pressure measurement depends on proper technique and equipment. Some key considerations include:

- Ensuring the cuff size is appropriate for the patient's arm circumference, as using a cuff that's too small or too large can result in inaccurate readings.

- Having the patient rest quietly for at least 5 minutes before taking a measurement.

- Placing the arm at heart level during measurement.

- Avoiding caffeine, exercise, and smoking for at least 30 minutes before measurement.

By understanding and properly applying these tools and techniques, healthcare providers and patients alike can ensure accurate blood pressure readings, which are essential for diagnosing hypertension and guiding its management. The subsequent sections will further explore the interpretation of these readings, the significance of blood pressure patterns, and how they influence the clinical approach to treating hypertension.

2.2 Interpreting Your Numbers

Understanding the numbers obtained from blood pressure measurements is crucial for both individuals and healthcare professionals. It not only aids in diagnosing hypertension but also in monitoring the effectiveness of treatments and lifestyle interventions. Blood pressure readings are represented by two numbers: the systolic pressure (the top number) and the diastolic pressure (the bottom number), measured in millimeters of mercury (mmHg).

Normal Blood Pressure: A reading of less than 120/80 mmHg is considered within the normal range. Individuals with blood pressure in this range should continue healthy lifestyle habits to maintain their blood pressure levels.

Elevated Blood Pressure: When readings consistently range from 120 to 129 systolic and less than 80 mmHg diastolic, the condition is classified as elevated blood pressure. This stage is a warning sign, indicating the need for lifestyle changes to prevent the development of hypertension.

Hypertension Stage 1: Blood pressure readings consistently ranging from 130 to 139 systolic or 80 to 89 diastolic are classified as stage 1 hypertension. At this stage, healthcare providers may recommend lifestyle modifications and possibly medication, based on the overall risk of cardiovascular disease.

Hypertension Stage 2: This stage is defined by systolic blood pressure of 140 mmHg or higher, or diastolic blood pressure of 90 mmHg or higher. Treatment typically involves a combination of medications and lifestyle changes.

Hypertensive Crisis: A systolic reading above 180 mmHg or a diastolic reading above 120 mmHg indicates a hypertensive crisis, requiring immediate medical attention. Symptoms may include severe headaches, shortness of breath, nosebleeds, or severe anxiety. This condition can lead to stroke, heart attack, kidney damage, or loss of consciousness.

Interpreting blood pressure numbers in the context of individual health profiles is essential. Factors such as age, family history of cardiovascular disease, presence of conditions like diabetes or chronic kidney disease, and overall cardiovascular risk should influence how blood pressure readings are interpreted and what treatment strategies are employed.

Monitoring Changes Over Time: Blood pressure can fluctuate throughout the day due to various factors, including activity levels, stress, and diet. Therefore, a single reading does not necessarily provide a complete picture of one's cardiovascular health. Regular monitoring can help identify patterns and trends, offering more insight into an individual's blood pressure profile and the effectiveness of treatment strategies.

Understanding your blood pressure numbers and what they represent empowers you to take an active role in managing your health. It is a crucial step towards preventing the complications associated with hypertension and achieving optimal cardiovascular health. Regular consultation with healthcare professionals can provide guidance tailored to individual needs and circumstances, ensuring that blood pressure management is both effective and sustainable.

2.3 When to Seek Medical Advice

Navigating the decision to seek medical advice for blood pressure concerns is a critical aspect of managing your overall health. Recognizing the signs that warrant professional evaluation can lead to early intervention, preventing the escalation of potential health issues. This section outlines scenarios and symptoms that should prompt you to consult a healthcare provider.

Consistently Elevated Blood Pressure Readings: If home monitoring or readings from pharmacy machines consistently show elevated blood pressure (systolic BP between 120-129 mmHg and diastolic less than 80 mmHg) or hypertension (systolic BP of 130 mmHg or higher, or diastolic BP of 80 mmHg or higher), it's important to seek medical advice. Early intervention can prevent the progression to more severe hypertension and reduce the risk of cardiovascular diseases.

Experiencing Symptoms of Hypertensive Crisis: A hypertensive crisis, characterized by systolic blood pressure over 180 mmHg or diastolic blood pressure over 120 mmHg, may sometimes manifest with acute symptoms. These can include severe headaches, chest pain, shortness of breath, severe anxiety, nosebleeds, or vision changes. Immediate medical attention is required as this condition can lead to organ damage or life-threatening complications.

Significant Lifestyle Change or New Diagnosis: If you're considering a significant lifestyle change, have recently been diagnosed with a condition that may affect your blood pressure (e.g., diabetes, kidney disease), or are planning to start a family, consulting with a healthcare provider can offer guidance tailored to your specific needs and health status.

Assessment of Blood Pressure Management Plan: For individuals already diagnosed with hypertension and undergoing treatment, regular medical reviews are crucial. These consultations help assess the effectiveness of current management plans, including medication efficacy, and adjust treatment as necessary based on changes in health status, blood pressure readings, or the development of side effects.

Before Starting New Medications or Supplements: Certain medications, over-the-counter drugs, and supplements can influence blood pressure. Before starting any new medication or supplement, consult a healthcare provider, especially if you have a history of hypertension or other cardiovascular conditions.

Pregnancy: Blood pressure management during pregnancy is critical, as hypertension can affect both the mother and the developing fetus. Women with pre-existing hypertension or those who develop hypertension during pregnancy should seek specialized care to manage their condition safely throughout pregnancy and postpartum.

Family History of Hypertension or Heart Disease: Individuals with a family history of hypertension or cardiovascular disease may have a higher risk of developing these conditions. Discussing your family health history with a healthcare provider can help in assessing your risk and determining a proactive health monitoring and management plan.

Seeking medical advice when necessary is a proactive step towards maintaining cardiovascular health and preventing the complications associated with uncontrolled blood pressure. Regular check-ups and open communication with healthcare providers ensure that any concerns are addressed promptly, allowing for timely adjustments to your health management strategy.

2.4 Exercise: 10 MCQs with Answers at the End

Test your knowledge on diagnosing hypertension with these multiple-choice questions. After completing the questions, check your answers at the end to see how well you've understood the concepts.

1. **What is the primary tool used to measure blood pressure in a clinical setting?**

   A. Stethoscope

   B. Sphygmomanometer

   C. Electrocardiogram (ECG)

   D. Treadmill

2. **Automated blood pressure monitors use which method to measure blood pressure?**

   A. Auscultatory method

   B. Oscillometric method

C. Palpatory method

D. Percussion method

3. What does Ambulatory Blood Pressure Monitoring (ABPM) help to identify?

A. Blood pressure variability over 24 hours

B. Immediate response to stress

C. Long-term cardiac health

D. Fitness level

4. Why is home blood pressure monitoring recommended?

A. It replaces the need for professional healthcare advice

B. To detect "white-coat hypertension"

C. To assess the effectiveness of blood pressure medications

D. All of the above

5. A hypertensive crisis is indicated by a systolic blood pressure over:

A. 120 mmHg

B. 140 mmHg

C. 160 mmHg

D. 180 mmHg

6. **Which factor does not affect the accuracy of blood pressure readings?**

A. Time of day

B. Arm position

C. Color of the blood pressure cuff

D. Cuff size

7. **Before measuring blood pressure, individuals should avoid which of the following for at least 30 minutes?**

A. Drinking water

B. Exercise

C. Sleeping

D. Reading

8. **Elevated blood pressure is defined as systolic readings:**

A. Below 120 mmHg

B. Between 120-129 mmHg and diastolic less than 80 mmHg

C. Above 130 mmHg

D. None of the above

9. **Seeking medical advice for hypertension is crucial when:**

A. Blood pressure is consistently above normal ranges

B. Experiencing symptoms of a hypertensive crisis

C. Starting new medications or supplements

D. All of the above

10. **Which is not a reason for regular medical review for individuals with hypertension?**

A. To socialize with healthcare providers

B. To adjust treatment based on current blood pressure readings

C. To assess the effectiveness of the management plan

D. To monitor for side effects of medications

Answers:

1. **B. Sphygmomanometer**

2. **B. Oscillometric method**

3. **A. Blood pressure variability over 24 hours**

4. **C. To assess the effectiveness of blood pressure medications**

5. **D. 180 mmHg**

6. **C. Color of the blood pressure cuff**

7. **B. Exercise**

8. **B. Between 120-129 mmHg and diastolic less than 80 mmHg**

9. **D. All of the above**

10. **A. To socialize with healthcare providers**

Chapter 3: The Impact of Lifestyle

3.1 Diet's Role in Blood Pressure Management

Diet plays a crucial role in the management and prevention of hypertension. It is one of the key lifestyle factors that can be adjusted to significantly impact blood pressure levels. A heart-healthy diet can help lower blood pressure, reduce the risk of developing hypertension, and support overall cardiovascular health.

Reduce Sodium Intake: Sodium is a major contributor to high blood pressure in many individuals. The body uses sodium to control blood volume and blood pressure. However, too much sodium causes the body to retain water, increasing blood volume and, consequently, blood pressure. Reducing sodium intake can significantly lower blood pressure levels. The American Heart Association recommends no more than 2,300 milligrams a day and moving toward an ideal limit of no more than 1,500 mg per day for most adults.

Increase Potassium Intake: Potassium helps balance the amount of sodium in your cells. A diet rich in potassium can help to lower blood pressure by easing tension in your blood vessel walls and helping to rid the body of excess sodium. Foods high in potassium include leafy greens, tomatoes, potatoes, sweet potatoes, fruit from vines (such as grapes and blackberries), root vegetables, and bananas.

DASH Diet: The Dietary Approaches to Stop Hypertension (DASH) diet is a well-researched dietary pattern designed to lower blood pressure. It emphasizes fruits, vegetables, whole grains, and lean proteins, including fish, poultry, beans, nuts, and vegetable oils. The DASH diet also limits foods high in saturated fat, such as fatty meats and full-fat dairy products, and it recommends cutting back on sugar-sweetened beverages and sweets.

Limit Alcohol and Caffeine: Alcohol can raise blood pressure by several points. It can also reduce the effectiveness of blood pressure medications. Limiting alcohol intake can help to keep your blood pressure in check. Similarly, caffeine can cause a short-term spike in blood pressure, although its long-term effects on blood pressure are less clear. Moderate coffee consumption (1-2 cups per day) seems to be heart-healthy for most people, but it's important to monitor your body's response.

Healthy Weight: Maintaining a healthy weight is an essential part of managing blood pressure. Excess weight forces your heart to work harder to pump blood to the body, which can raise your blood pressure. Losing even a small amount of weight if you're overweight or obese can help reduce your blood pressure. In general, you may reduce your blood pressure by about 1 mm Hg for every kilogram (about 2.2 pounds) of weight you lose.

Balanced Diet: A balanced diet that includes a variety of foods rich in nutrients, fiber, and healthy fats can support heart health and blood pressure management. Incorporate a variety of fruits, vegetables, whole grains, and lean protein sources into your diet to maximize the benefits.

Incorporating these dietary changes into your lifestyle can have a profound effect on your blood pressure and overall health. It's not about a short-term diet but rather a long-term dietary pattern that promotes heart health. Consulting with a healthcare provider or a dietitian can provide personalized advice and support to help you make the necessary adjustments to your diet for effective blood pressure management.

3.2 Exercise and Physical Activity

Exercise and physical activity are fundamental elements in the management and prevention of hypertension, offering a multitude of benefits for cardiovascular health. Regular physical activity strengthens the heart, enabling it to pump more blood with less effort. As the heart becomes more efficient, the force on the arteries decreases, lowering blood pressure. This chapter delves into how incorporating exercise into your routine can aid in controlling hypertension and outlines strategies for getting started.

Types of Exercise Beneficial for Lowering Blood Pressure:

- **Aerobic Exercise:** Activities such as walking, jogging, cycling, swimming, or dancing can significantly lower blood pressure by improving heart and lung fitness. Aim for at least 150 minutes of moderate-intensity aerobic activity or 75 minutes of vigorous-intensity activity per week, as recommended by the American Heart Association.

- **Resistance Training:** Moderate resistance training (e.g., using weights, resistance bands, or body weight) two or three days a week can also help reduce blood pressure by increasing muscle strength and endurance. It's important to focus on major muscle groups and to avoid holding your breath during these exercises, as this can temporarily increase blood pressure.

- **Dynamic Resistance Exercises:** Exercises that involve movements of muscles through their full range of motion, such as squats, leg presses, or arm curls, can be particularly effective. These exercises help improve flexibility, balance, and strength.

- **High-intensity Interval Training (HIIT):** HIIT involves short bursts of intense activity alternated with periods of lighter activity or rest. This type of training can be efficient in improving cardiovascular fitness and reducing blood pressure within a shorter timeframe, making it a good option for those with busy schedules.

Getting Started with Exercise:

1. **Consult with a Healthcare Provider:** Before starting any new exercise program, especially if you have been diagnosed with hypertension or have other health concerns, it's crucial to consult with a healthcare provider. They can offer guidance tailored to your health status and fitness level.

2. **Start Slowly:** If you're new to exercise or have been inactive, start with shorter sessions of moderate activity and gradually increase the duration and intensity as your fitness improves.

3. **Incorporate Physical Activity into Daily Life:** Besides structured exercise, look for ways to incorporate more physical activity into your day, such as taking the stairs instead of the elevator, walking or biking instead of driving for short distances, or standing up and moving around during breaks if you have a sedentary job.

4. **Set Realistic Goals:** Setting achievable goals can help you stay motivated. Celebrate your progress, no matter how small, and adjust your goals as your fitness level improves.

5. **Find Activities You Enjoy:** Exercise should be something you look forward to, not dread. Experiment with different activities to find what you enjoy most, and consider varying your routine to keep it interesting.

Monitoring Your Blood Pressure:

- As you incorporate exercise into your lifestyle, continue to monitor your blood pressure regularly. This will allow you to see the positive effects of physical activity on your blood pressure and help you stay motivated.

- Pay attention to how your body responds during and after exercise. If you experience any discomfort or symptoms such as dizziness, chest pain, or shortness of breath, stop the activity immediately and seek medical advice.

Regular physical activity is a powerful tool in the fight against hypertension. By making exercise a regular part of your life, you can significantly improve your heart health, lower your blood pressure, and reduce your risk of cardiovascular disease.

3.3 Stress Management Techniques

Stress plays a significant role in hypertension. While short-term stress can cause temporary spikes in blood pressure, chronic stress can lead to long-term blood pressure issues, partly through the unhealthy habits people adopt in an attempt to manage stress, such as eating high-sodium comfort foods, drinking alcohol, or smoking. Effective stress management is, therefore, an integral part of blood pressure control. This section explores various techniques to help manage and reduce stress, contributing to overall well-being and lower blood pressure levels.

Mindfulness and Meditation: Mindfulness meditation involves focusing your mind on the present moment, acknowledging and accepting your feelings, thoughts, and bodily sensations. Regular practice can help reduce stress, lower blood pressure, and improve overall heart health. Even a few minutes a day can make a significant difference.

Deep Breathing Exercises: Deep breathing techniques, such as abdominal breathing and focused breathing, can help activate the body's relaxation response, reducing stress and lowering blood pressure. Practice deep breathing for a few minutes each day, especially during moments of heightened stress.

Physical Activity: Exercise is not only crucial for maintaining physical health but also for stress reduction. Physical activity increases the production of endorphins, the brain's feel-good neurotransmitters, and can act as a form of meditation in motion, helping to clear the mind and relieve tension.

Yoga and Tai Chi: Yoga combines physical postures, breathing exercises, meditation, and a distinct philosophy to promote physical and mental well-being. Tai Chi, a form of martial arts known for its health benefits, involves gentle movements and deep breaths to reduce stress and anxiety. Both practices are effective for stress management and blood pressure reduction.

Time Management: Poor time management can lead to stress, rushing from one task to another, and feeling perpetually behind. Learning to prioritize tasks, saying no when necessary, and setting aside time for relaxation and hobbies can help reduce stress levels.

Social Support: Having a strong network of friends and family can provide emotional support and a sense of belonging, reducing stress. Spending time with loved ones or participating in group activities can be an effective way to relax and de-stress.

Professional Help: When stress becomes overwhelming, seeking the help of a psychologist or professional counselor can be beneficial. Cognitive-behavioral therapy (CBT) and other counseling techniques can provide strategies to manage stress more effectively.

Healthy Sleep Habits: Adequate sleep is essential for stress management. Develop a regular sleep routine, create a comfortable sleep environment, and avoid stimulants such as caffeine close to bedtime to improve sleep quality.

Relaxation Techniques: Techniques such as progressive muscle relaxation, guided imagery, and biofeedback can help reduce muscle tension and stress. These practices involve systematically relaxing different muscle groups in the body and visualizing peaceful scenes or situations.

Incorporating these stress management techniques into your daily routine can help mitigate the effects of stress on your blood pressure and overall health. While it's not always possible to eliminate stress from your life, developing healthy coping mechanisms can significantly reduce its impact on your well-being.

3.4 Exercise: 10 MCQs with Answers at the End

Evaluate your understanding of the impact of lifestyle on blood pressure management with these multiple-choice questions. Check your answers at the end to see how well you've grasped the key concepts.

1. **Regular physical activity can lower blood pressure by:**

   A. Increasing heart rate

   B. Strengthening the heart muscle

   C. Narrowing the arteries

   D. Increasing body weight

2. **The DASH diet specifically recommends:**

   A. High sodium intake

   B. High fat intake

C. Increased fruits and vegetables

D. Exclusive protein consumption

3. **Mindfulness meditation aids in blood pressure management by:**

A. Ignoring current stressors

B. Focusing on the past

C. Focusing on the present moment

D. Planning for future events

4. **Which of the following is not a recommended stress management technique?**

A. Deep breathing exercises

B. Regular consumption of alcohol

C. Yoga

D. Tai Chi

5. **Effective time management can reduce stress by:**

A. Increasing the number of tasks to complete

B. Prioritizing tasks

C. Eliminating all leisure activities

D. Working without breaks

6. **Potassium helps to manage blood pressure by:**

   A. Increasing sodium levels in the body

   B. Reducing tension in blood vessel walls

   C. Decreasing heart muscle strength

   D. Promoting water retention

7. **The primary benefit of aerobic exercise in hypertension management is:**

   A. Reducing cognitive function

   B. Improving lung capacity only

   C. Improving heart and lung fitness

   D. Increasing stress levels

8. **Social support may aid in stress management by:**

   A. Isolating individuals from friends

   B. Providing emotional support and a sense of belonging

   C. Increasing dependence on others

   D. Reducing the need for professional help

9. **A diet low in sodium is important for managing hypertension because sodium:**

   A. Strengthens the heart muscle

   B. Helps the body eliminate excess fluid

C. Causes the body to retain water, increasing blood volume

D. Reduces potassium levels in the body

10. Which of the following is a benefit of good sleep habits for blood pressure management?

A. Increased stress and anxiety

B. Elevated nighttime blood pressure

C. Reduced stress and improved relaxation

D. Increased caffeine sensitivity

Answers:

1. **B. Strengthening the heart muscle**

2. **C. Increased fruits and vegetables**

3. **C. Focusing on the present moment**

4. **B. Regular consumption of alcohol**

5. **B. Prioritizing tasks**

6. **B. Reducing tension in blood vessel walls**

7. **C. Improving heart and lung fitness**

8. **B. Providing emotional support and a sense of belonging**

9. **C. Causes the body to retain water, increasing blood volume**

10. **C. Reduced stress and improved relaxation**

Chapter 4: Medical Management of Hypertension

4.1 First-Line Hypertension Medications

The medical management of hypertension often involves the use of medications to lower blood pressure, reduce the risk of cardiovascular disease, and prevent the complications associated with high blood pressure. First-line hypertension medications are those typically recommended to start treatment, based on their effectiveness, safety profile, and the ability to reduce cardiovascular risks. This section outlines the common classes of first-line medications for treating hypertension.

Angiotensin-Converting Enzyme (ACE) Inhibitors: ACE inhibitors work by blocking the conversion of angiotensin I to angiotensin II, a potent vasoconstrictor. This action relaxes blood vessels and lowers blood pressure. Examples include lisinopril, enalapril, and ramipril. They are particularly effective in patients with diabetes, chronic kidney disease, or a history of heart failure.

Angiotensin II Receptor Blockers (ARBs): ARBs block the action of angiotensin II, leading to vasodilation and reduced blood pressure. They offer a similar benefit to ACE inhibitors but with a lower risk of certain side effects, such as cough. Examples include losartan, valsartan, and olmesartan.

Calcium Channel Blockers (CCBs): CCBs inhibit the entry of calcium into the cells of the heart and blood vessels, which relaxes the blood vessels and reduces blood pressure. They are particularly useful in older adults and those of African descent. Examples include amlodipine, diltiazem, and verapamil.

Thiazide Diuretics: Thiazide diuretics help the kidneys remove sodium and water from the body, which lowers blood volume and reduces blood pressure. They have been shown to prevent cardiovascular events and are cost-effective. Examples include hydrochlorothiazide and chlorthalidone.

Beta-Blockers: Beta-blockers reduce blood pressure by slowing the heart rate and reducing the heart's workload. While they are not always the first choice for initial treatment of hypertension, they are particularly beneficial for patients with certain conditions, such as ischemic heart disease or heart failure. Examples include metoprolol, atenolol, and bisoprolol.

It's important to note that the choice of medication may depend on individual patient characteristics, including age, race, and the presence of other medical conditions. For example, ACE inhibitors and ARBs are often preferred in patients with diabetes due to their protective effects on the kidneys.

Combination Therapy: Many patients with hypertension may require more than one medication to achieve blood pressure goals. Combination therapy using medications from different classes can be more effective than increasing the dose of a single medication. Fixed-dose combination pills, which contain two or more medications, can simplify the regimen and improve adherence.

Managing hypertension is a personalized process, and medication needs may change over time. Regular follow-up with a healthcare provider is essential to monitor blood pressure, assess the effectiveness of the treatment, and make adjustments as needed. Lifestyle changes, such as diet and exercise, remain an important part of managing hypertension, even when medications are prescribed.

4.2 Understanding Side Effects

While first-line hypertension medications are effective in managing high blood pressure and reducing the risk of cardiovascular complications, like all medications, they can have side effects. Understanding these side effects is crucial for patients to manage their treatment effectively and maintain their quality of life. This section provides an overview of common side effects associated with various classes of hypertension medications and strategies for managing them.

Angiotensin-Converting Enzyme (ACE) Inhibitors:

- **Common Side Effects:** Dry cough, increased blood potassium levels (hyperkalemia), fatigue, dizziness, and in rare cases, angioedema (swelling of the deep layers of the skin).

- **Management Strategies:** If a dry cough develops, an Angiotensin II Receptor Blocker (ARB) may be used as an alternative. Monitoring potassium levels and renal function is also important.

Angiotensin II Receptor Blockers (ARBs):

- **Common Side Effects:** Dizziness, hyperkalemia, and occasional drowsiness or fatigue.

- **Management Strategies:** Similar to ACE inhibitors, monitoring potassium levels is important. Staying hydrated and standing up slowly can help reduce dizziness.

Calcium Channel Blockers (CCBs):

- **Common Side Effects:** Swelling of the feet and lower legs (peripheral edema), constipation (particularly with verapamil), dizziness, and palpitations.

- **Management Strategies:** Elevating the legs can help with edema. Including fiber in the diet can prevent constipation. If side effects persist, consulting with a healthcare provider for a possible change in medication may be necessary.

Thiazide Diuretics:

- **Common Side Effects:** Electrolyte imbalances (such as low potassium levels), increased blood sugar levels, increased uric acid levels, and in some cases, erectile dysfunction.

- **Management Strategies:** Regular blood tests to monitor electrolytes and glucose levels are important. Potassium supplements or a potassium-rich diet may be recommended if levels are low.

Beta-Blockers:

- **Common Side Effects:** Fatigue, cold hands and feet, slow heartbeat, and symptoms of asthma or chronic obstructive pulmonary disease (COPD) in susceptible individuals. Some may also experience sleep disturbances or depression.

- **Management Strategies:** Taking the medication at night may help reduce daytime fatigue. Beta-blockers that are more cardio-selective may have fewer respiratory side effects and are preferred in patients with lung conditions.

General Strategies for Managing Side Effects:

- **Open Communication:** Always inform your healthcare provider about any side effects you experience. There may be alternative medications or dosages that can reduce side effects.

- **Lifestyle Modifications:** Some side effects can be managed with lifestyle changes, such as diet modifications for constipation or exercise for fatigue.

- **Medication Timing:** Taking medications at specific times of the day can sometimes help minimize side effects. For example, diuretics taken in the morning can prevent nocturnal bathroom visits.

Understanding and managing the side effects of hypertension medications is a collaborative process between the patient and healthcare provider. With careful monitoring and open communication, most side effects can be effectively managed, allowing patients to continue their treatment while maintaining a good quality of life.

4.3 Monitoring and Adjusting Treatment

Effective management of hypertension requires ongoing monitoring and, sometimes, adjustments to the treatment plan. This process ensures that blood pressure goals are met and maintained over time, minimizing the risk of cardiovascular complications. Here's how patients and healthcare providers can work together to monitor and adjust hypertension treatment as needed.

Regular Blood Pressure Monitoring:

- **At Home:** Patients are often encouraged to monitor their blood pressure at home using a validated blood pressure monitor. This provides valuable information about how blood pressure varies throughout the day and in different settings.

- **In the Clinic:** Regular check-ups with a healthcare provider are essential for assessing blood pressure control and evaluating the effectiveness of the treatment plan.

Assessing Medication Effectiveness and Side Effects:

- During follow-up appointments, healthcare providers will review the effectiveness of prescribed medications and inquire about any side effects experienced. It's crucial for patients to communicate openly about their experiences, including adherence to the medication regimen and any challenges faced.

Adjusting Medication Dosage or Regimen:

- Based on the monitoring results and patient feedback, adjustments to the medication dosage or regimen may be necessary. This could involve increasing the dose of a current medication, adding a new medication to the regimen, or switching to a different medication if side effects are problematic.

Lifestyle Modification Review:

- In addition to medication, lifestyle modifications play a crucial role in managing hypertension. Healthcare providers will review and reinforce the importance of a healthy diet, regular physical activity, weight management, smoking cessation, and limited alcohol consumption. Adjustments to these lifestyle factors may be recommended based on the patient's progress and current health status.

Special Considerations:

- **Resistant Hypertension:** Some patients may have resistant hypertension, meaning their blood pressure remains high despite being on three different blood pressure-lowering medications, including a diuretic. In such cases, further evaluation and more complex treatment strategies may be necessary.

- **Secondary Hypertension:** If blood pressure is difficult to control or there is a sudden onset of high blood pressure, healthcare providers may investigate for secondary causes of hypertension, such as kidney disease or hormonal disorders.

Patient Education and Empowerment:

- Educating patients about the importance of monitoring, treatment adherence, and lifestyle changes is key to successful hypertension management. Empowering patients with knowledge and resources helps them to take an active role in their treatment.

Regular Follow-Up:

- Scheduling regular follow-up appointments is essential for ongoing assessment of blood pressure control, medication management, and lifestyle modifications. The frequency of these appointments will depend on the severity of hypertension, how well it's controlled, and any other underlying health conditions.

Effective management of hypertension is a dynamic process that requires collaboration between patients and healthcare providers. Through regular monitoring, open communication, and willingness to adjust treatment plans as needed, blood pressure can be effectively managed, reducing the risk of complications and improving overall health outcomes.

4.4 Exercise: 10 MCQs with Answers at the End

Test your understanding of the medical management of hypertension with these multiple-choice questions. Refer to the answers at the end for self-assessment.

1. What class of medication is typically a first-line treatment for hypertension?

A. ACE Inhibitors

B. Antidepressants

C. Antihistamines

D. Antifungals

2. Which medication works by blocking the effects of angiotensin II?

A. Calcium Channel Blockers

B. Angiotensin II Receptor Blockers (ARBs)

C. Beta-Blockers

D. Diuretics

3. What is a common side effect of ACE inhibitors?

A. Dry cough

B. Increased hair growth

C. Weight gain

D. Night vision improvement

4. Which of the following is a lifestyle change recommended in conjunction with medication for managing hypertension?

A. Increasing sodium intake

B. Reducing physical activity

C. Limiting alcohol consumption

D. Increasing caffeine intake

5. What does resistant hypertension mean?

A. Blood pressure that is too low

B. Blood pressure that is controlled with a single medication

C. Blood pressure that remains high despite taking three different medications

D. Blood pressure that fluctuates frequently

6. **Calcium Channel Blockers are particularly useful for patients in which demographic?**

A. Young adults

B. Athletes

C. Older adults and those of African descent

D. Children under 12

7. **Which technique is NOT a method of monitoring blood pressure?**

A. Using a sphygmomanometer

B. Measuring waist circumference

C. Home blood pressure monitoring

D. Ambulatory Blood Pressure Monitoring (ABPM)

8. **Beta-Blockers may cause which of the following side effects?**

A. Slow heartbeat

B. Sudden increase in energy

C. Decrease in cholesterol levels

D. Improved sense of smell

9. **For a patient with diabetes and hypertension, which class of medication might be particularly beneficial?**

   A. ACE Inhibitors or ARBs

   B. Antipsychotics

   C. Oral contraceptives

   D. Anabolic steroids

10. **Thiazide diuretics help lower blood pressure by:**

   A. Increasing blood volume

   B. Slowing down heart rate

   C. Removing sodium and water from the body

   D. Blocking calcium channels

Answers:

1. **A. ACE Inhibitors**

2. **B. Angiotensin II Receptor Blockers (ARBs)**

3. **A. Dry cough**

4. **C. Limiting alcohol consumption**

5. **C. Blood pressure that remains high despite taking three different medications**

6. **C. Older adults and those of African descent**

7. **B. Measuring waist circumference**

8. **A. Slow heartbeat**

9. **A. ACE Inhibitors or ARBs**

10. **C. Removing sodium and water from the body**

Chapter 5: Alternative Therapies and Remedies

5.1 Herbal and Natural Supplements

In the management of hypertension, many individuals seek out herbal and natural supplements as complementary or alternative options to conventional medication. While some of these supplements have been studied for their potential blood pressure-lowering effects, it's important to approach them with caution, understanding their benefits and risks, and always discussing their use with a healthcare provider before starting. Here's a look at some commonly considered supplements:

Garlic: Studies have shown that garlic, particularly in its aged form, may have a modest blood pressure-lowering effect due to its ability to help relax blood vessels. However, the amount needed to achieve a therapeutic effect might exceed what can be consumed through diet alone.

Omega-3 Fatty Acids: Found in fish oil and flaxseeds, omega-3 fatty acids are known for their heart health benefits, including potentially lowering blood pressure. They may help reduce inflammation and thin the blood, improving cardiovascular health.

Hibiscus Tea: Consumed in many cultures for its health benefits, hibiscus tea has been found in some studies to lower systolic and diastolic blood pressure. Its effects are thought to be similar to some ACE inhibitors, relaxing the arteries and reducing fluid retention.

Magnesium: This mineral helps regulate blood pressure by relaxing blood vessels. While magnesium supplements may benefit those with a deficiency or specific health conditions, getting magnesium through a balanced diet is generally preferred.

Potassium: Like magnesium, potassium helps balance the amount of sodium in your body and eases tension in your blood vessel walls. While supplements are available, it's often recommended to increase potassium intake through diet (fruits, vegetables, dairy) unless otherwise advised by a healthcare provider.

Coenzyme Q10 (CoQ10): CoQ10 is an antioxidant that has been studied for its potential to lower blood pressure. While some research suggests a benefit, more studies are needed to confirm its effectiveness and optimal dosing.

Green Tea: Known for its antioxidant properties, green tea may also help lower blood pressure, although evidence is mixed. Moderate consumption is generally considered safe and potentially beneficial for heart health.

Cautions and Considerations:

- **Interactions with Medications:** Herbal supplements can interact with prescription medications, either enhancing or diminishing their effects. It's crucial to consult with a healthcare provider before combining supplements with medications.

- **Quality and Dosage:** The quality and potency of herbal supplements can vary widely between products. Opt for brands that have been independently tested for quality and purity.

- **Underlying Conditions:** Some supplements may not be suitable for individuals with certain health conditions or those undergoing surgery.

While alternative therapies and remedies can complement traditional hypertension management, they should not replace prescribed medications without the guidance of a healthcare provider. A holistic approach that includes lifestyle changes, medication as needed, and possibly supplements, under professional supervision, can provide the best strategy for managing high blood pressure.

5.2 Acupuncture and Pressure Points

Acupuncture, a key component of traditional Chinese medicine, has been explored as a potential treatment for various conditions, including hypertension. It involves the insertion of very thin needles through the skin at strategic points on the body. The practice is based on the belief that this can balance the body's energy flow or Qi (pronounced "chee") and, consequently, improve health.

Acupuncture for Hypertension:

- **Mechanism:** The proposed mechanisms by which acupuncture might lower blood pressure include promoting relaxation and reducing stress, thus decreasing sympathetic nervous system activity, which is known to raise blood pressure. Additionally, it's thought to stimulate the release of endorphins and other neurohumoral factors, influencing the body's homeostatic mechanisms.

- **Evidence:** Clinical studies on acupuncture's effectiveness for hypertension have yielded mixed results. Some research suggests that acupuncture can lead to modest reductions in blood pressure in patients with hypertension, particularly when combined with other treatments or lifestyle modifications. However, other studies have not found significant benefits, leading to ongoing debate about its effectiveness for this purpose.

- **Treatment Approach:** When used for hypertension, acupuncture treatment typically focuses on specific points believed to influence cardiovascular health. Common points include PC6, LI11, ST36, and LR3. The selection of points may vary based on the individual's condition and the acupuncturist's assessment.

Pressure Points and Massage:

- **Acupressure:** Similar to acupuncture, acupressure involves the application of pressure to specific points on the body. It can be performed by a practitioner or as self-care and may help manage stress and reduce blood pressure.

- **Massage Therapy:** Massage therapy, particularly techniques that promote relaxation and reduce stress, may have a beneficial effect on blood pressure. Regular sessions can help lower stress levels, potentially impacting blood pressure over time.

Considerations:

- **Professional Guidance:** It's essential to seek treatment from a licensed and experienced acupuncturist or massage therapist who is familiar with managing hypertension.

- **Integration with Conventional Care:** Acupuncture and pressure points techniques should complement, not replace, conventional hypertension management, including medication and lifestyle changes.

- **Individual Response:** Response to these therapies can vary widely among individuals. Some may experience significant benefits, while others notice little change.

- **Safety and Side Effects:** Acupuncture is generally considered safe when performed by a trained professional, with minimal side effects. Common side effects include soreness, minor bleeding, or bruising at the needle sites.

While acupuncture and pressure point techniques offer potential benefits for blood pressure management, they are best utilized as part of a comprehensive approach that includes traditional medical treatment and lifestyle modifications. Discussing these options with a healthcare provider can ensure that they fit safely and effectively into your overall hypertension management plan.

5.3 Mind-Body Techniques

Mind-body techniques encompass a variety of practices that use the mind's ability to affect physical health. These techniques have been increasingly recognized for their potential in managing hypertension, as they address the stress and emotional factors that can influence blood pressure. Here's an overview of some mind-body approaches that may benefit individuals with hypertension:

Meditation: Meditation, including mindfulness meditation, transcendental meditation, and other forms, encourages focused attention and awareness. Regular meditation has been shown to reduce stress levels, which can help lower blood pressure. Studies suggest that consistent practice may lead to modest reductions in both systolic and diastolic blood pressure.

Yoga: Yoga combines physical postures, breathing exercises, and meditation or relaxation. It not only helps in reducing stress but also improves physical fitness. Certain yoga practices, particularly those emphasizing relaxation and breathing, have been found to have a positive effect on blood pressure.

Biofeedback: Biofeedback techniques enable individuals to gain control over certain bodily processes that are normally involuntary, such as heart rate, muscle tension, and blood pressure. By using sensors connected to a machine, users receive feedback that helps them learn to adjust these processes. Biofeedback has been used to manage hypertension by teaching individuals how to relax their muscles and reduce stress.

Progressive Muscle Relaxation (PMR): PMR involves sequentially tensing and then relaxing different muscle groups in the body. This practice promotes overall relaxation and has been found to lower stress and potentially reduce blood pressure.

Guided Imagery: This technique involves focusing the mind on peaceful, calming images and scenarios to reduce stress. Guided imagery can be done independently or with the help of recordings or a therapist. It's a simple, versatile tool for relaxation that can complement hypertension management.

Tai Chi and Qigong: These traditional Chinese practices combine slow, deliberate movements, meditation, and breathing exercises. They are known for reducing stress and have been studied for their potential in lowering blood pressure. Tai Chi and Qigong are particularly appealing for their gentle approach, making them suitable for individuals of all fitness levels.

Breathing Exercises: Deep breathing and controlled breathing practices can activate the body's relaxation response, helping to lower blood pressure. Techniques such as the "4-7-8" breathing method or abdominal breathing can be easily learned and practiced anywhere.

Considerations for Practice:

- **Consultation with Healthcare Providers:** Before starting any mind-body practice, particularly if you have hypertension or other health conditions, it's important to consult with healthcare providers. They can offer guidance on appropriate practices and any precautions.

- **Regular Practice:** Consistency is key to achieving the potential benefits of mind-body techniques. Regular, daily practice is often more effective than occasional use.

- **Integration with Conventional Treatment:** Mind-body techniques should complement, not replace, conventional hypertension treatments such as medication and lifestyle changes.

Mind-body techniques offer a promising adjunctive approach to hypertension management, with the potential to improve both mental and physical well-being. By incorporating these practices into a comprehensive care plan, individuals with hypertension can take an active role in managing their condition and enhancing their overall health.

5.4 Exercise: 10 MCQs with Answers at the End

Evaluate your knowledge on alternative therapies and remedies for hypertension with these multiple-choice questions. Check the answers provided at the end to see how well you understand the material.

1. **Garlic supplements are thought to lower blood pressure by:**

   A. Increasing heart rate

   B. Thinning the blood

   C. Relaxing blood vessels

   D. Decreasing heart muscle strength

2. **Which supplement is known for its heart health benefits, including potential blood pressure lowering effects?**

   A. Vitamin C

   B. Omega-3 Fatty Acids

   C. Calcium

   D. Vitamin D

3. **Hibiscus tea may lower blood pressure by mechanisms similar to:**

   A. Beta-Blockers

   B. ACE Inhibitors

   C. Calcium Channel Blockers

   D. Diuretics

4. **Which mineral helps regulate blood pressure by relaxing blood vessels?**

A. Iron

B. Magnesium

C. Zinc

D. Copper

5. **Mindfulness meditation aids in blood pressure management primarily through:**

A. Increasing physical activity

B. Reducing stress

C. Enhancing nutrient absorption

D. Strengthening heart muscle

6. **Yoga contributes to lower blood pressure by:**

A. Causing rapid weight loss

B. Improving lung capacity only

C. Reducing stress and improving physical fitness

D. Increasing sodium excretion

7. **Biofeedback helps individuals with hypertension by:**

A. Teaching them to control involuntary bodily processes

B. Increasing their metabolism

C. Directly reducing cholesterol levels

D. Altering their genetic predisposition to hypertension

8. Which of the following is NOT typically a benefit of practicing Tai Chi?

A. Enhanced muscular strength

B. Immediate cure for hypertension

C. Stress reduction

D. Improvement in balance and flexibility

9. Progressive Muscle Relaxation (PMR) works by:

A. Increasing heart rate variability

B. Tensing and then relaxing muscle groups

C. Promoting rapid, shallow breathing

D. Decreasing bone density

10. Guided Imagery is a technique that:

A. Requires advanced physical skills

B. Focuses the mind on peaceful images to reduce stress

C. Increases blood pressure through visualization

D. Involves high-intensity interval training

Answers:

1. **C. Relaxing blood vessels**

2. **B. Omega-3 Fatty Acids**

3. **B. ACE Inhibitors**

4. **B. Magnesium**

5. **B. Reducing stress**

6. **C. Reducing stress and improving physical fitness**

7. **A. Teaching them to control involuntary bodily processes**

8. **B. Immediate cure for hypertension**

9. **B. Tensing and then relaxing muscle groups**

10. **B. Focuses the mind on peaceful images to reduce stress**

Chapter 6: Hypertension in Special Populations

6.1 Children and Adolescents

Hypertension is not exclusive to adults; it can also affect children and adolescents. Recognizing and managing high blood pressure in these younger populations is crucial for preventing long-term health complications. This section explores the unique considerations, diagnosis, and management strategies for hypertension in children and adolescents.

Prevalence and Importance:

- Although less common than in adults, hypertension in children and adolescents is increasingly recognized, partly due to rising obesity rates. Early detection and management are vital to reduce the risk of cardiovascular disease later in life.

Risk Factors:

- **Obesity:** The most significant risk factor for pediatric hypertension. The prevalence of obesity in children and adolescents has increased dramatically, paralleling the rise in hypertension.

- **Family History:** Like adults, a family history of hypertension increases the risk in children.

- **Underlying Conditions:** Certain medical conditions, such as kidney disease, endocrine disorders, and congenital heart disease, can contribute to hypertension.

Diagnosis:

- Blood pressure measurements in children are interpreted differently than in adults, with normal values varying by age, sex, and height. Hypertension is diagnosed when a child's blood pressure is at or above the 95th percentile for their age, sex, and height on three or more occasions.

- The American Academy of Pediatrics (AAP) recommends routine blood pressure screenings for children starting at age 3 during annual wellness visits.

Management Strategies:

- **Lifestyle Modifications:** The first line of treatment involves lifestyle changes, such as increasing physical activity, adopting a healthy diet (similar to the DASH diet recommended for adults), and achieving a healthy weight.

- **Medication:** If lifestyle modifications are insufficient or if the child has symptomatic hypertension or secondary hypertension due to another condition, medication may be necessary. The choice of medication is similar to that in adults but adjusted for pediatric use.

Unique Considerations:

- **Growth and Development:** Treatment plans must consider the child's ongoing growth and development. Regular monitoring is essential to adjust medication dosages and ensure the treatment remains effective without adverse effects on growth.

- **Psychosocial Factors:** The psychological and social aspects of living with hypertension can significantly impact a child's or adolescent's quality of life, necessitating support from family, school, and healthcare providers.

Prevention:

- Preventive measures play a crucial role in addressing pediatric hypertension. Encouraging healthy eating habits, regular physical activity, and limiting screen time are key strategies to prevent high blood pressure from developing in the first place.

Conclusion:

Hypertension in children and adolescents requires a comprehensive approach that includes early detection, lifestyle modifications, possible pharmacological treatment, and ongoing monitoring. By addressing hypertension early, it's possible to mitigate its impact and reduce the risk of cardiovascular disease in adulthood. Collaboration among healthcare providers, parents, and schools is essential to support the health and well-being of children and adolescents with hypertension.

6.2 Pregnancy-Induced Hypertension

Pregnancy-induced hypertension (PIH), also known as gestational hypertension, is a condition characterized by high blood pressure that develops after the 20th week of pregnancy in women who previously had normal blood pressure. Recognizing and managing PIH is crucial for the health of both the mother and the fetus, as it can lead to complications such as preeclampsia, a more severe condition associated with serious health risks.

Prevalence and Importance:

- PIH affects approximately 6-8% of pregnant women. It's important to differentiate between gestational hypertension and preeclampsia, as the latter includes the presence of protein in the urine and more severe complications.

Risk Factors:

- **First Pregnancy:** The risk of PIH is higher in a woman's first pregnancy.

- **History of Hypertension or PIH:** Women with a history of hypertension or previous PIH have an increased risk.

- **Multiple Pregnancy:** The risk increases with twin or multiple pregnancies.

- **Maternal Age:** Both teenage and women over 40 are at increased risk.

- **Underlying Health Conditions:** Pre-existing conditions such as kidney disease, diabetes, or autoimmune diseases.

- **Obesity:** Higher body mass index (BMI) before pregnancy.

Diagnosis:

- PIH is diagnosed when a pregnant woman has a blood pressure reading of 140/90 mmHg or higher on two occasions, at least four hours apart, after 20 weeks of pregnancy without the presence of protein in the urine.

Management Strategies:

- **Monitoring:** Regular monitoring of blood pressure and urine protein levels is essential for early detection and management.

- **Lifestyle Modifications:** While specific lifestyle modifications for PIH are limited during pregnancy, maintaining a healthy diet and staying physically active as recommended by a healthcare provider can be beneficial.

- **Medication:** In some cases, antihypertensive medications may be prescribed to manage blood pressure during pregnancy. The choice of medication is carefully considered to ensure safety for both the mother and the fetus.

- **Delivery Planning:** In cases where PIH develops into preeclampsia or if there are signs of fetal distress, early delivery may be recommended to prevent complications.

Complications:

- Without proper management, PIH can progress to preeclampsia, characterized by proteinuria and more severe symptoms, including liver or renal dysfunction, severe headaches, visual disturbances, and edema. Preeclampsia requires immediate medical attention to prevent eclampsia, a life-threatening condition.

Prevention:

- There is no definitive way to prevent PIH, but regular prenatal care allows for early detection and management. For women with a history of PIH or at high risk, low-dose aspirin starting after the first trimester may be recommended as a preventive measure.

Conclusion:

Pregnancy-induced hypertension demands careful monitoring and management to safeguard the health of both the mother and the baby. Through regular prenatal care, early detection, and appropriate treatment, the risks associated with PIH can be significantly reduced, leading to healthier outcomes for both mother and child. Collaboration between obstetricians, midwives, and primary care providers is essential in providing comprehensive care to pregnant women with hypertension.

6.3 The Elderly and Hypertension

Hypertension is a prevalent condition among the elderly, affecting a significant proportion of individuals over the age of 65. Managing high blood pressure in this population presents unique challenges and considerations, given the presence of coexisting medical conditions, the increased risk of cardiovascular events, and the potential for adverse effects from treatment.

Prevalence and Importance:

- The prevalence of hypertension increases with age, partly due to changes in vascular structure and function. In the elderly, hypertension is a major risk factor for stroke, heart disease, kidney failure, and cognitive decline.

Risk Factors:

- **Aging Process:** Natural changes in blood vessel elasticity and function contribute to increased blood pressure.

- **Lifestyle Factors:** Sedentary lifestyle, poor diet, and excess salt intake, common among some elderly populations, exacerbate hypertension risk.

- **Coexisting Conditions:** Conditions like diabetes, obesity, and renal disease, more common in older adults, increase the complexity of hypertension management.

Diagnosis:

- Blood pressure targets and treatment thresholds may be adjusted in elderly patients, considering overall health, life expectancy, and potential benefits versus risks of treatment. The decision to treat and the blood pressure goals are individualized based on patient-specific factors.

Management Strategies:

- **Lifestyle Modifications:** Encouraging a heart-healthy diet, regular physical activity, and weight management remains fundamental. Modifications should be realistic and consider the physical and cognitive abilities of the elderly individual.

- **Medication:** The selection of antihypertensive medication in the elderly should take into account the presence of other medical conditions, the risk of interactions with other medications, and the potential for side effects. Lower initial doses and gradual titration may help minimize adverse effects.

- **Polypharmacy:** Many elderly patients are on multiple medications, increasing the risk of drug-drug interactions and side effects. Regular review of all medications is essential to manage polypharmacy effectively.

Unique Considerations in the Elderly:

- **Orthostatic Hypotension:** A drop in blood pressure upon standing can be more common in the elderly, especially with certain antihypertensive drugs. Monitoring for symptoms and adjusting treatment as needed is important.

- **Cognitive Function:** Blood pressure management should consider its impact on cognitive function, with both hypertension and certain antihypertensive medications potentially affecting cognition.

- **Frailty and Falls:** Treatment plans should balance the benefits of blood pressure control with the risk of falls and injuries, particularly in frail elderly patients.

Conclusion:

Managing hypertension in the elderly requires a careful, personalized approach that balances the benefits of blood pressure reduction with the potential risks of treatment. Lifestyle modifications, appropriate selection and dosing of medications, and regular monitoring are key components of effective management. Involvement of caregivers and a multidisciplinary healthcare team can support the comprehensive care needed to optimize outcomes in elderly individuals with hypertension.

6.4 Exercise: 10 MCQs with Answers at the End

Test your knowledge on hypertension in special populations with these multiple-choice questions. Check your answers at the end to gauge your understanding of the material.

1. What is a significant risk factor for developing hypertension in children and adolescents?

A. High protein diet

B. Excessive water intake

C. Obesity

D. Insufficient sunlight exposure

2. Pregnancy-induced hypertension typically develops after how many weeks of pregnancy?

A. 10 weeks

B. 20 weeks

C. 30 weeks

D. 40 weeks

3. Which of the following is NOT a common risk factor for hypertension in the elderly?

A. Increased vascular stiffness

B. Sedentary lifestyle

C. High potassium diet

D. Coexisting conditions like diabetes

4. First-line treatment for hypertension in children often involves:

A. Immediate initiation of medication

B. Lifestyle modifications

C. Surgical intervention

D. Herbal supplements

5. Preeclampsia is a condition associated with:

A. Diabetes mellitus

B. Pregnancy-induced hypertension

C. Chronic kidney disease

D. Atherosclerosis

6. **An important consideration in treating hypertension in the elderly is:**

A. The potential for rapid progression

B. Minimizing physical activity to reduce strain

C. The risk of orthostatic hypotension

D. Increasing sodium intake to maintain electrolyte balance

7. **Low-dose aspirin in pregnancy is recommended for:**

A. All pregnant women

B. Those with a history of PIH or at high risk

C. Pregnant women over 35

D. Women with low blood pressure

8. **Management of hypertension in children and adolescents focuses primarily on:**

A. Lifestyle modifications and, if necessary, medication

B. Aggressive medication regimen

C. Bloodletting

D. High-sodium diet to increase blood volume

9. **In managing hypertension, why is polypharmacy a concern for the elderly?**

   A. It increases physical fitness

   B. It reduces cognitive function

   C. It raises the risk of drug-drug interactions and side effects

   D. It significantly decreases blood pressure

10. **Regular prenatal care is essential for managing PIH because it allows for:**

   A. Early delivery planning

   B. Avoidance of all medications

   C. Increased physical activity

   D. Consumption of herbal supplements

Answers:

1. **C. Obesity**

2. **B. 20 weeks**

3. **C. High potassium diet**

4. **B. Lifestyle modifications**

5. **B. Pregnancy-induced hypertension**

6. **C. The risk of orthostatic hypotension**

7. **B. Those with a history of PIH or at high risk**

8. **A. Lifestyle modifications and, if necessary, medication**

9. **C. It raises the risk of drug-drug interactions and side effects**

10. **A. Early delivery planning**

Chapter 7: Complications of Uncontrolled Hypertension

7.1 Heart Disease and Stroke

Uncontrolled hypertension, or high blood pressure, is a leading risk factor for cardiovascular diseases, including heart disease and stroke. The relentless pressure exerted against the artery walls can lead to various forms of heart disease, while also significantly increasing the risk of stroke. Understanding these complications is crucial for appreciating the importance of managing blood pressure.

Heart Disease:

- **Coronary Artery Disease (CAD):** Hypertension can lead to the hardening and narrowing of the arteries (atherosclerosis), reducing blood flow to the heart muscle and potentially resulting in chest pain (angina), heart attack, or heart failure.

- **Left Ventricular Hypertrophy (LVH):** The increased workload on the heart caused by high blood pressure can cause the heart's main pumping chamber (left ventricle) to thicken and stiffen, impairing the heart's ability to pump blood efficiently. LVH is a significant predictor of heart failure and sudden cardiac death.

- **Heart Failure:** Over time, the strain hypertension places on the heart can weaken the heart muscle, leading to heart failure, a condition where the heart can't pump enough blood to meet the body's needs.

Stroke:

- **Ischemic Stroke:** The most common type of stroke, occurring when a blood vessel supplying blood to the brain is obstructed, often by a blood clot. Hypertension is a major risk factor for the development of the atherosclerotic plaques that can lead to these clots.

- **Hemorrhagic Stroke:** High blood pressure can cause blood vessels in the brain to weaken, leading to a burst or bleed. This type of stroke can be particularly devastating and is more directly linked to high blood pressure than ischemic strokes.

Prevention and Management:

- **Blood Pressure Control:** Effectively managing blood pressure through lifestyle changes and medication can significantly reduce the risk of heart disease and stroke.

- **Healthy Lifestyle:** A diet low in salt and saturated fats, regular physical activity, maintaining a healthy weight, and avoiding tobacco use can help lower blood pressure and reduce cardiovascular risk.

- **Regular Monitoring:** For individuals with hypertension, regular monitoring of blood pressure and heart health, including the use of echocardiograms to detect LVH and other potential issues, is crucial.

Conclusion:

The link between uncontrolled hypertension and the risk of heart disease and stroke underscores the critical importance of managing blood pressure. By adopting a comprehensive approach to blood pressure control, including lifestyle modifications and medical management, individuals can significantly reduce their risk of these life-threatening complications. Regular check-ups and collaboration with healthcare providers are essential to tailor the management plan to individual needs and to adjust treatment as necessary to achieve optimal blood pressure control.

7.2 Kidney Damage and Failure

Uncontrolled hypertension is a leading cause of kidney damage and failure, underscoring the critical connection between blood pressure management and kidney health. The kidneys play a vital role in filtering waste from the blood and regulating blood pressure, fluid balance, and electrolyte levels. High blood pressure can harm the kidneys' blood vessels, diminishing their filtering capabilities and leading to long-term damage.

Kidney Damage:

- **Nephrosclerosis:** Chronic hypertension can lead to the hardening and narrowing of the blood vessels in the kidneys (arteriosclerosis), reducing blood flow. This condition, known as nephrosclerosis, can gradually impair kidney function.

- **Glomerular Damage:** High blood pressure can damage the glomeruli, the tiny filtering units within the kidneys, affecting their ability to filter waste effectively. Over time, this damage can lead to proteinuria (protein in the urine) and a decline in kidney function.

Kidney Failure:

- **Chronic Kidney Disease (CKD):** Persistent kidney damage can progress to CKD, a condition characterized by a gradual loss of kidney function over time. Early stages may be asymptomatic or present minimal symptoms, making regular screening important for those with hypertension.

- **End-Stage Renal Disease (ESRD):** In its advanced stages, CKD can evolve into ESRD, requiring dialysis or a kidney transplant for survival. Hypertension is a significant risk factor for the progression to ESRD.

Prevention and Management:

- **Blood Pressure Control:** Effective management of hypertension is crucial for preventing kidney damage. Target blood pressure levels may be lower for individuals with kidney disease, as recommended by healthcare providers.

- **Lifestyle Modifications:** Diet, exercise, and weight management play essential roles in both blood pressure and kidney health. Reducing salt intake and limiting foods high in animal proteins and saturated fats can be beneficial.

- **Medication:** Certain antihypertensive medications, such as ACE inhibitors and ARBs, not only help control blood pressure but also have protective effects on the kidneys by reducing proteinuria and slowing the progression of kidney damage.

- **Regular Monitoring:** Individuals with hypertension should undergo regular kidney function tests, including serum creatinine, estimated glomerular filtration rate (eGFR), and urine albumin-to-creatinine ratio (ACR), to detect early signs of kidney impairment.

Conclusion:

The relationship between uncontrolled hypertension and kidney damage emphasizes the importance of diligent blood pressure management to preserve kidney health. By implementing a comprehensive approach that includes lifestyle changes, medication, and regular monitoring, individuals with hypertension can significantly reduce their risk of kidney-related complications. Collaboration with healthcare providers is essential to customize the treatment plan, monitor kidney function, and adjust strategies as needed to protect against kidney damage and failure.

7.3 Vision Loss and Eye Damage

Uncontrolled hypertension can have profound effects on the eyes, leading to conditions that may cause vision loss and irreversible eye damage. High blood pressure can damage the delicate vessels in the retina, the part of the eye responsible for capturing light and sending visual signals to the brain. This section discusses the impact of hypertension on eye health and strategies for prevention and management.

Hypertensive Retinopathy:

- **Definition:** A condition characterized by damage to the retina caused by high blood pressure. It can lead to blurred vision, eye bleeding, and, in severe cases, blindness.

- **Symptoms:** Often, there are no early symptoms. As the condition progresses, symptoms might include visual disturbances, headaches, and vision loss.

Choroidopathy:

- **Definition:** This condition involves the accumulation of fluid under the retina due to a leaky blood vessel in the layer of blood vessels located under the retina, known as the choroid. It can result in distorted or impaired vision.

- **Symptoms:** Symptoms may include distorted vision where straight lines appear wavy, as well as scotomas or blind spots.

Optic Neuropathy:

- **Definition:** High blood pressure can lead to blocked blood flow to the optic nerve, causing optic neuropathy. This can result in severe, sudden vision loss.

- **Symptoms:** Symptoms include sudden vision loss in one or both eyes, sometimes accompanied by pain on movement of the affected eye(s).

Prevention and Management:

- **Blood Pressure Control:** Effective control of hypertension is crucial for preventing eye damage. Regular monitoring and treatment, including lifestyle modifications and medications, can help maintain blood pressure within a healthy range.

- **Regular Eye Exams:** Routine eye exams are essential for detecting early signs of damage to the retina or other parts of the eye. Early detection allows for timely treatment to prevent progression.

- **Manage Overall Cardiovascular Health:** Managing other risk factors for cardiovascular disease, such as diabetes, high cholesterol, and smoking, is also important for eye health.

- **Prompt Treatment of Hypertensive Episodes:** Managing episodes of severely elevated blood pressure promptly can prevent acute damage to the eyes and other organs.

Conclusion:

The potential for hypertension to cause vision loss and eye damage highlights the importance of comprehensive blood pressure management and regular eye care. By taking steps to control blood pressure and by monitoring eye health regularly, individuals with hypertension can significantly reduce their risk of hypertensive retinopathy and other eye-related complications. Collaboration between healthcare providers, including primary care physicians and ophthalmologists, is essential to ensure an integrated approach to the management of hypertension and the prevention of related eye conditions.

7.4 Exercise: 10 MCQs with Answers at the End

Assess your understanding of the complications associated with uncontrolled hypertension with these multiple-choice questions. Refer to the answers provided at the end for self-assessment.

1. **Hypertensive retinopathy is primarily caused by damage to the:**

   A. Optic nerve

   B. Retina

   C. Lens

   D. Cornea

2. **Which condition involves the accumulation of fluid under the retina due to hypertension?**

   A. Glaucoma

   B. Choroidopathy

   C. Cataract

   D. Macular degeneration

3. **Sudden vision loss from hypertension may indicate:**

A. Optic neuropathy

B. Hyperopia

C. Astigmatism

D. Presbyopia

4. **A significant risk factor for chronic kidney disease (CKD) progression in hypertensive patients is:**

A. Low sodium diet

B. Excessive exercise

C. Uncontrolled high blood pressure

D. High potassium intake

5. **Coronary artery disease (CAD) in hypertensive patients can lead to all EXCEPT:**

A. Angina

B. Heart attack

C. Heart failure

D. Hyperopia

6. **Left Ventricular Hypertrophy (LVH) caused by hypertension results in:**

   A. Weakening of the heart's right chamber

   B. Thinning of the heart's walls

   C. Thickening and stiffening of the heart's left chamber

   D. Increased flexibility of the heart's valves

7. **The primary mechanism through which hypertension leads to stroke is by:**

   A. Increasing cerebral oxygen demand

   B. Causing dehydration

   C. Damaging blood vessels in the brain

   D. Reducing glucose levels in the brain

8. **Management of hypertensive retinopathy focuses on:**

   A. Direct treatment of the retina

   B. Laser eye surgery

   C. Control of hypertension

   D. Immediate use of corrective lenses

9. **Which of the following is NOT a direct complication of uncontrolled hypertension?**

A. Stroke

B. Retinopathy

C. Myopia

D. Kidney failure

10. **Preventing end-stage renal disease (ESRD) in hypertensive patients involves:**

A. Ignoring proteinuria

B. Strict control of blood pressure

C. Avoiding all medications

D. Consuming high-sodium foods

Answers:

1. **B. Retina**

2. **B. Choroidopathy**

3. **A. Optic neuropathy**

4. **C. Uncontrolled high blood pressure**

5. **D. Hyperopia**

6. **C. Thickening and stiffening of the heart's left chamber**

7. **C. Damaging blood vessels in the brain**

8. **C. Control of hypertension**

9. **C. Myopia**

10. **B. Strict control of blood pressure**

Chapter 8: Diet and Nutrition

8.1 Salt and Its Effects

Salt, specifically its sodium component, plays a significant role in the regulation of blood pressure. While sodium is an essential nutrient required for bodily functions, including nerve transmission and muscle contraction, excessive intake can lead to an increase in blood pressure, posing risks for hypertension and related health complications. Understanding the effects of salt on blood pressure and overall health is crucial for managing dietary intake and reducing hypertension risk.

How Salt Affects Blood Pressure:

- **Fluid Retention:** Sodium attracts and holds water. High sodium intake causes the body to retain extra fluid, increasing the volume of blood in the bloodstream, which can raise blood pressure.

- **Increased Cardiac Load:** The added blood volume from high sodium intake forces the heart to work harder and places more pressure on the arteries, contributing to hypertension.

- **Vascular Resistance:** Over time, high salt intake may contribute to the stiffening of blood vessels, increasing resistance to blood flow and further elevating blood pressure.

Recommended Sodium Intake:

- The American Heart Association recommends limiting sodium intake to less than 2,300 milligrams (mg) a day, with an ideal limit of no more than 1,500 mg per day for most adults, especially those with hypertension or at risk of developing high blood pressure.

Sources of Dietary Sodium:

- **Processed and Packaged Foods:** A significant portion of dietary sodium comes from processed foods, such as canned soups, frozen dinners, and packaged snacks.

- **Restaurant Meals:** Meals eaten out, including fast food, often contain high levels of sodium.

- **Table Salt:** While table salt is an obvious source, it accounts for only a small percentage of total sodium intake for most people.

Strategies to Reduce Sodium Intake:

- **Read Labels:** Pay attention to the sodium content on food labels and choose lower-sodium options.

- **Prepare Meals at Home:** Cooking at home allows for better control over sodium levels in food.

- **Use Herbs and Spices:** Flavor food with herbs, spices, and citrus instead of salt.

- **Choose Fresh or Frozen Produce:** Opt for fresh or frozen fruits and vegetables over canned varieties, which often contain added salt.

- **Limit Processed Foods:** Reduce consumption of processed and packaged foods, which are common sources of added sodium.

Health Benefits of Reducing Sodium Intake:

- Lowering sodium intake can help reduce blood pressure in individuals with hypertension and those at risk of developing high blood pressure. It can also decrease the risk of heart disease, stroke, and kidney damage.

Conclusion:

Modifying dietary sodium intake is a key strategy in managing hypertension and improving cardiovascular health. By understanding the sources of sodium and adopting strategies to limit its consumption, individuals can make significant strides in controlling their blood pressure and reducing the risk of hypertension-related complications.

8.2 Potassium's Role in Control

Potassium is a vital mineral that plays a significant role in managing blood pressure and maintaining overall cardiovascular health. It works in concert with sodium to regulate water balance, nerve signals, and muscle contractions in the body. Understanding potassium's role and how to incorporate it effectively into the diet can significantly aid in blood pressure control.

How Potassium Affects Blood Pressure:

- **Balancing Sodium:** Potassium helps balance the amount of sodium in your cells. High sodium levels can raise blood pressure, but potassium helps the kidneys excrete excess sodium, thus lowering blood pressure.

- **Relaxing Blood Vessels:** Potassium aids in the relaxation of blood vessel walls, which can help reduce blood pressure by decreasing vascular resistance.

Recommended Potassium Intake:

- The American Heart Association suggests an intake of at least 4,700 milligrams (mg) of potassium per day for adults. This recommendation is based on the benefits of potassium in counteracting the effects of sodium and reducing blood pressure.

Dietary Sources of Potassium:

- **Fruits:** Bananas, oranges, cantaloupe, honeydew, apricots, grapefruit (some citrus fruits should be consumed with caution if taking specific blood pressure medications)

- **Vegetables:** Potatoes, tomatoes, sweet potatoes, green leafy vegetables (spinach, kale), and cucumbers

- **Beans and Legumes:** Lentils, kidney beans, soybeans, and white beans

- **Nuts and Seeds:** Almonds, peanuts, and sunflower seeds

- **Dairy:** Milk and yogurt are good sources of potassium

- **Fish:** Salmon, tuna, and halibut

Considerations When Increasing Potassium Intake:

- **Kidney Function:** Individuals with kidney disease need to be cautious with potassium intake, as impaired kidneys may not be able to remove excess potassium from the blood, potentially leading to hyperkalemia (high blood potassium levels).

- **Medication Interactions:** Some blood pressure medications, like ACE inhibitors and ARBs, can increase potassium levels in the blood. It's important to monitor potassium intake if you're taking these medications.

Strategies to Increase Potassium Intake:

- **Incorporate Potassium-rich Foods:** Aim to include a variety of potassium-rich foods in your diet, focusing on whole foods like fruits, vegetables, and legumes.

- **Limit Processed Foods:** Processed and packaged foods are not only high in sodium but often low in potassium. Opting for fresh or minimally processed foods can help increase your potassium intake.

- **Consult a Healthcare Provider:** If you have conditions that affect potassium metabolism, such as kidney disease, or if you're on blood pressure medication, consult with your healthcare provider to determine the right potassium intake level for you.

Conclusion:

Potassium is an essential nutrient that can help lower blood pressure and mitigate the adverse effects of high sodium intake. By incorporating potassium-rich foods into the diet and considering individual health needs and medication interactions, individuals can effectively manage their blood pressure and contribute to overall cardiovascular health.

8.3 Managing Calories and Weight

Effective management of calories and maintaining a healthy weight are crucial components in controlling hypertension. Excess body weight increases the risk of high blood pressure by enhancing vascular resistance and placing additional strain on the heart. By managing caloric intake and striving for a healthy weight, individuals can significantly lower their blood pressure and reduce the risk of cardiovascular complications.

The Relationship Between Weight and Blood Pressure:

- Excess body weight can lead to increased blood volume and pressure on artery walls, contributing to higher blood pressure.

- Obesity is also associated with insulin resistance, which can further elevate blood pressure by increasing sodium retention and sympathetic nervous system activity.

Caloric Management for Weight Loss:

- **Understanding Caloric Needs:** Daily caloric needs vary based on age, sex, weight, height, and level of physical activity. Utilizing online calculators or consulting with a healthcare provider can help determine your specific caloric needs for weight maintenance or loss.

- **Caloric Deficit for Weight Loss:** To lose weight, individuals must consume fewer calories than they expend. A deficit of 500 to 1,000 calories per day can lead to a safe weight loss of about 1 to 2 pounds per week.

Dietary Strategies for Weight and Blood Pressure Control:

- **Reduce Processed and High-Calorie Foods:** Limiting foods high in processed sugars, saturated fats, and empty calories can reduce overall caloric intake and support weight loss.

- **Increase Fruits, Vegetables, and Whole Grains:** These foods are not only lower in calories but also high in fiber, vitamins, and minerals, which can help manage hunger and support overall health.

- **Portion Control:** Being mindful of portion sizes can help control caloric intake without the need for drastic dietary changes.

Physical Activity:

- Regular physical activity is essential for creating a caloric deficit and promoting weight loss. Activities such as walking, cycling, swimming, and strength training not only burn calories but also improve cardiovascular health.

- The American Heart Association recommends at least 150 minutes of moderate-intensity aerobic activity or 75 minutes of vigorous-intensity activity per week, plus muscle-strengthening activities on 2 or more days per week.

Monitoring Progress:

- Keeping track of weight, dietary intake, and physical activity can help individuals stay accountable and make adjustments as needed.

- Regular check-ups with a healthcare provider can provide additional support and guidance.

Conclusion:

Managing calories and weight is a foundational strategy in the control of hypertension. By adopting a balanced diet, practicing portion control, and engaging in regular physical activity, individuals can effectively reduce their blood pressure and enhance their overall cardiovascular health. It's important to approach weight loss and caloric management as long-term lifestyle changes rather than short-term diets for sustained health benefits.

8.4 Exercise: 10 MCQs with Answers at the End

Evaluate your understanding of diet, nutrition, and their impact on hypertension with these multiple-choice questions. Review the answers provided at the end for self-assessment.

1. **Excessive sodium intake affects blood pressure by:**

A. Decreasing heart rate

B. Increasing fluid retention

C. Lowering blood volume

D. Reducing vascular resistance

2. The recommended daily potassium intake for adults is at least:

A. 2,300 mg

B. 3,500 mg

C. 4,700 mg

D. 5,200 mg

3. A healthy weight loss rate per week is:

A. 0.5 to 1 pound

B. 1 to 2 pounds

C. 3 to 4 pounds

D. 5 to 6 pounds

4. Which of the following dietary approaches is specifically recommended for hypertension management?

A. Keto diet

B. Paleo diet

C. DASH diet

D. Atkins diet

5. **Regular physical activity contributes to blood pressure management by:**

A. Increasing sodium retention

B. Decreasing heart and lung fitness

C. Lowering heart rate and improving vessel flexibility

D. Promoting weight gain

6. **Processed and packaged foods are known to be high in:**

A. Potassium

B. Dietary fiber

C. Sodium

D. Vitamins

7. **Which of the following is a benefit of reducing caloric intake and losing weight?**

A. Increased blood pressure

B. Reduced vascular resistance

C. Higher cholesterol levels

D. Decreased insulin sensitivity

8. **Omega-3 fatty acids are beneficial for heart health because they:**

A. Increase LDL cholesterol

B. Reduce inflammation and blood clotting

C. Elevate blood pressure

D. Decrease HDL cholesterol

9. **A dietary strategy for managing hypertension includes:**

A. Adding extra salt to meals

B. Increasing consumption of processed foods

C. Reducing intake of fruits and vegetables

D. Limiting alcohol consumption

10. **Effective weight management for hypertension involves:**

A. Ignoring physical activity recommendations

B. Consuming a high-sodium diet

C. Creating a caloric deficit through diet and exercise

D. Focusing solely on rapid weight loss methods

Answers:

1. **B. Increasing fluid retention**

2. **C. 4,700 mg**

3. **B. 1 to 2 pounds**

4. **C. DASH diet**

5. **C. Lowering heart rate and improving vessel flexibility**

6. **C. Sodium**

7. **B. Reduced vascular resistance**

8. **B. Reduce inflammation and blood clotting**

9. **D. Limiting alcohol consumption**

10. **C. Creating a caloric deficit through diet and exercise**

Chapter 9: Physical Activity and Exercise

9.1 Building an Effective Exercise Regimen

Incorporating regular physical activity into your daily routine is a key strategy in managing hypertension and improving overall cardiovascular health. An effective exercise regimen can help lower blood pressure, reduce stress, and enhance heart function. This section provides guidance on how to create a balanced and sustainable exercise program.

Assessing Fitness Level:

- Before starting any new exercise regimen, evaluate your current fitness level. Consider factors like how often you currently exercise, what activities you engage in, and your comfort level with different forms of exercise.

- Consulting with a healthcare provider is crucial, especially if you have been diagnosed with hypertension or other health conditions. They can recommend safe starting points and necessary precautions.

Setting Realistic Goals:

- Establish clear, achievable goals based on your health status, lifestyle, and preferences. Whether it's lowering blood pressure, losing weight, or improving endurance, having specific objectives can keep you motivated.

- Start with manageable targets, such as walking for 30 minutes a day, and gradually increase intensity or duration as your fitness improves.

Incorporating Various Types of Exercise:

- **Aerobic Exercise:** Activities like walking, jogging, cycling, swimming, and dancing are effective at improving heart and lung fitness, lowering blood pressure, and burning calories. Aim for at least 150 minutes of moderate-intensity or 75 minutes of high-intensity aerobic exercise per week.

- **Strength Training:** Building muscle through resistance training (e.g., weightlifting, bodyweight exercises) at least two days a week can help reduce fat mass, increase metabolism, and support overall health. Ensure proper form and technique to avoid injury.

- **Flexibility and Stretching:** Incorporating flexibility exercises or stretching into your routine can improve range of motion, reduce the risk of injury, and promote muscle relaxation.

- **Balance Training:** As you age, balance exercises become increasingly important to prevent falls and maintain physical independence. Practices such as yoga or Tai Chi are beneficial for enhancing balance.

Listening to Your Body:

- Monitor how your body responds to exercise, especially if you're managing hypertension. If you experience symptoms such as dizziness, chest pain, or excessive fatigue, adjust your activity level and consult your healthcare provider.

Maintaining Consistency and Motivation:

- Finding activities you enjoy is key to sustaining an exercise regimen. Experiment with different types of exercise to keep your routine interesting and engaging.

- Regularly tracking your progress, setting new goals, and rewarding yourself for achievements can help maintain motivation.

Staying Safe:

- Warm up before and cool down after exercise to prepare your muscles and reduce the risk of injury.

- Stay hydrated, especially during intense or prolonged physical activity.

- Wear appropriate footwear and clothing to support your activities and protect against environmental factors.

Conclusion:

Building an effective exercise regimen is a cornerstone of managing hypertension and promoting cardiovascular health. By assessing your fitness level, setting realistic goals, incorporating a variety of exercises, and listening to your body's signals, you can create a sustainable and beneficial physical activity routine that supports your health objectives. Regular consultation with healthcare providers ensures that your exercise program aligns with your medical needs and health goals.

9.2 Cardiovascular vs. Strength Training

Both cardiovascular (cardio) and strength training exercises play crucial roles in managing hypertension and enhancing overall health, but they offer different benefits. Understanding the distinctions and complementary nature of these two types of exercise can help you create a balanced fitness regimen that effectively addresses blood pressure management and cardiovascular health.

Cardiovascular Training:

- **Definition and Examples:** Cardiovascular or aerobic exercise involves sustained physical activity that increases heart and lung fitness. Examples include walking, jogging, cycling, swimming, and rowing.

- **Benefits for Hypertension:** Cardio exercises are particularly effective at lowering blood pressure and improving heart health. They increase heart rate and enhance the heart's efficiency, leading to improved circulation and reduced strain on the cardiovascular system.

- **Frequency and Duration:** The American Heart Association recommends at least 150 minutes of moderate-intensity aerobic activity or 75 minutes of vigorous-intensity activity per week, spread throughout the week.

Strength Training:

- **Definition and Examples:** Strength training, or resistance training, involves exercises that improve muscle strength and endurance. This can be achieved using free weights, weight machines, resistance bands, or body weight exercises like push-ups and squats.

- **Benefits for Hypertension:** While the immediate effect of strength training on blood pressure can vary, regular practice contributes to weight loss, increased muscle mass, and improved metabolic health, all of which can help lower blood pressure over time. It also strengthens the musculoskeletal system, improving overall functionality and independence, especially in older adults.

- **Frequency and Guidelines:** It's recommended to engage in muscle-strengthening activities targeting all major muscle groups on two or more days a week, with at least 48 hours of rest between sessions for any given muscle group.

Integrating Cardio and Strength Training:

- **Balanced Approach:** For optimal health benefits, including blood pressure management, a fitness regimen should include both cardio and strength training. Balancing these exercises can help ensure comprehensive health benefits, covering cardiovascular, musculoskeletal, and metabolic health.

- **Customization Based on Health Goals:** The ratio of cardio to strength training can be adjusted based on personal health goals, preferences, and medical advice. For instance, someone focusing on weight loss might prioritize cardio, while someone aiming to build muscle mass might increase strength training sessions.

- **Adaptation Over Time:** As fitness levels improve, the intensity and variety of exercises can be adjusted to continue challenging the body, promoting further improvements in health and well-being.

Safety Considerations:

- Individuals with hypertension should monitor their blood pressure response to different types of exercise, particularly when starting a new fitness regimen or significantly changing their exercise routine.

- Consultation with healthcare providers before starting or modifying exercise programs is essential to ensure safety and effectiveness, especially for those with existing health conditions.

Conclusion:

Cardiovascular and strength training exercises offer complementary benefits for managing hypertension and improving cardiovascular health. A well-rounded fitness regimen that includes both types of exercise, tailored to individual health goals and conditions, can provide the most comprehensive health benefits. Regular consultation with healthcare professionals ensures that exercise choices align with personal health needs and contribute positively to managing hypertension.

9.3 Exercise Precautions and Safety

While exercise is a key component of managing hypertension and promoting overall health, certain precautions are necessary to ensure safety, especially for those with high blood pressure or other medical conditions. Understanding and adhering to these precautions can help prevent adverse effects and maximize the benefits of physical activity.

Consultation with a Healthcare Provider:

- Before starting any new exercise program, it's crucial for individuals with hypertension or other health concerns to consult with their healthcare provider. This consultation can help determine the types and intensity levels of exercise that are safe and beneficial.

Start Slowly and Progress Gradually:

- For those not accustomed to regular physical activity, it's important to start with low-intensity exercises and gradually increase intensity and duration over time. This approach helps the body adapt safely without placing undue strain on the heart and blood vessels.

Monitor Blood Pressure:

- Individuals with hypertension should monitor their blood pressure in response to exercise, especially when making changes to their exercise regimen. This monitoring can help identify how different types of physical activity affect blood pressure and adjust as needed.

Stay Hydrated:

- Adequate hydration is important before, during, and after exercise. Dehydration can affect blood pressure and overall performance, so it's important to drink water regularly throughout physical activities.

Warm-Up and Cool-Down:

- Incorporating warm-up and cool-down periods before and after exercise sessions can help prevent sudden changes in blood pressure. Warm-up exercises gradually increase heart rate and prepare the muscles for activity, while cool-down exercises help gradually return the body to its resting state.

Be Aware of Environmental Conditions:

- Extreme temperatures and high humidity can affect blood pressure and the body's ability to regulate temperature. It's advisable to exercise indoors in controlled environments when outdoor conditions are harsh or to adjust the intensity and duration of outdoor workouts accordingly.

Recognize Signs of Overexertion:

- Symptoms such as dizziness, chest pain, excessive shortness of breath, palpitations, or feeling faint are warning signs of overexertion. If these symptoms occur, stop the activity immediately and seek medical advice if necessary.

Use Proper Equipment and Technique:

- Using appropriate exercise equipment and maintaining correct form and technique can help prevent injuries and ensure the effectiveness of the workout. This is particularly important for strength training exercises.

Avoid Valsalva Maneuver:

- The Valsalva maneuver, which involves holding the breath and straining during exertion (common in weightlifting), can cause a sudden increase in blood pressure. It's important to breathe regularly throughout each exercise to avoid this risk.

Incorporate Variety:

- A varied exercise program that includes aerobic, strength, flexibility, and balance activities not only enhances overall fitness but also reduces the risk of overuse injuries and keeps the regimen engaging.

Conclusion:

By following these exercise precautions and safety guidelines, individuals with hypertension can enjoy the health benefits of physical activity while minimizing potential risks. Regular consultation with healthcare providers is essential to tailor exercise programs to individual health needs and conditions, ensuring that physical activity remains a safe and effective part of hypertension management.

9.4 Exercise: 10 MCQs with Answers at the End

Test your knowledge on physical activity and exercise precautions for hypertension with these multiple-choice questions. Check your answers at the end to assess your understanding.

1. Before starting a new exercise regimen, individuals with hypertension should first:

A. Increase their salt intake

B. Consult with a healthcare provider

C. Start with high-intensity exercises

D. Purchase expensive exercise equipment

2. Gradual progression in exercise is important to:

A. Quickly reduce blood pressure to normal levels

B. Prevent boredom during workouts

C. Safely adapt the body to increased activity

D. Increase muscle mass within a few days

3. **Monitoring blood pressure in response to exercise helps to:**

   A. Decrease the effectiveness of workouts

   B. Understand how different activities affect blood pressure

   C. Increase blood pressure variability

   D. Reduce the need for hypertension medication

4. **Proper hydration during exercise is important because dehydration can:**

   A. Lower blood pressure too much

   B. Improve cardiovascular endurance

   C. Affect blood pressure and overall performance

   D. Increase muscle flexibility

5. **A warm-up period before exercising is important to:**

   A. Reduce the total time spent on workouts

   B. Prevent sudden changes in blood pressure

   C. Increase the chance of muscle injury

   D. Decrease the body's temperature

6. **When exercising in extreme temperatures or high humidity, it's advisable to:**

   A. Ignore the weather conditions

   B. Extend the workout duration

C. Adjust the intensity and duration accordingly

D. Focus solely on hydration

7. Symptoms such as dizziness and chest pain during exercise are signs of:

A. Adequate intensity

B. Overexertion

C. Effective weight loss

D. Increased muscle strength

8. Using appropriate equipment and maintaining correct form during exercise helps to:

A. Make workouts easier

B. Prevent injuries and ensure workout effectiveness

C. Decrease the duration of each workout session

D. Eliminate the need for a cool-down period

9. The Valsalva maneuver during exercise can cause:

A. A sudden decrease in blood pressure

B. A sudden increase in blood pressure

C. Improved cardiovascular health

D. Longer endurance

10. **A varied exercise program includes:**

A. Only aerobic exercises

B. Only high-intensity interval training

C. Aerobic, strength, flexibility, and balance activities

D. Solely balance exercises for elderly individuals

Answers:

1. **B. Consult with a healthcare provider**

2. **C. Safely adapt the body to increased activity**

3. **B. Understand how different activities affect blood pressure**

4. **C. Affect blood pressure and overall performance**

5. **B. Prevent sudden changes in blood pressure**

6. **C. Adjust the intensity and duration accordingly**

7. **B. Overexertion**

8. **B. Prevent injuries and ensure workout effectiveness**

9. **B. A sudden increase in blood pressure**

10. **C. Aerobic, strength, flexibility, and balance activities**

Chapter 10: Stress Management

10.1 Understanding the Stress Response

The stress response, often referred to as "fight or flight," is the body's automatic, built-in system designed to protect us from threat or harm. While stress is a normal part of life, chronic stress, especially without effective management, can have significant health implications, including the development or exacerbation of hypertension. Understanding how the stress response works can help in identifying strategies for managing stress and minimizing its impact on blood pressure.

The Physiology of Stress:

- **Activation of the Sympathetic Nervous System:** When faced with a perceived threat, the sympathetic nervous system is activated, releasing stress hormones like adrenaline and cortisol. These hormones increase heart rate, elevate blood pressure, and boost energy supplies.

- **Short-Term Responses:** Initially, these physiological changes are beneficial, preparing the body to either confront or flee from danger. They enhance focus, energy, and strength.

- **Chronic Stress:** If the stress response is activated frequently or if stressors persist over time without adequate recovery, the body remains in a state of heightened alert. Chronic activation of the stress response can lead to health issues, including persistent hypertension, anxiety, depression, digestive problems, and sleep disturbances.

Impact of Chronic Stress on Blood Pressure:

- Chronic stress can lead to sustained high blood pressure as the body continuously releases stress hormones, keeping blood vessels in a more constricted state.

- Over time, chronic stress can also contribute to other behaviors that increase the risk of hypertension, such as unhealthy eating habits, physical inactivity, and smoking.

Managing the Stress Response:

- **Recognition:** The first step in managing stress is recognizing its signs and symptoms, such as irritability, anxiety, sleep problems, and changes in appetite.

- **Healthy Lifestyle Choices:** Engaging in regular physical activity, maintaining a balanced diet, getting adequate sleep, and practicing relaxation techniques can help mitigate the effects of stress.

- **Stress Reduction Techniques:** Techniques such as deep breathing, meditation, yoga, and mindfulness can activate the body's relaxation response, counteracting the effects of stress.

- **Social Support:** Building and maintaining a supportive network of friends and family can provide emotional support and help in coping with stress.

- **Professional Help:** For those struggling to manage stress on their own, seeking help from a mental health professional can provide strategies to cope more effectively.

Conclusion:

Understanding the stress response and its impact on health is crucial for developing effective stress management strategies. By recognizing stress triggers, adopting healthy lifestyle habits, and utilizing stress reduction techniques, individuals can better manage their stress levels, potentially reducing the risk or severity of hypertension. Regular consultation with healthcare professionals can also provide additional support and guidance tailored to individual needs.

10.2 Techniques for Reducing Stress

Effectively managing stress is crucial for maintaining both mental and physical health, including the regulation of blood pressure. Various techniques can be employed to reduce stress, each offering different benefits. By integrating these practices into daily life, individuals can find relief from stress and its negative impact on health, including hypertension.

Deep Breathing Exercises:

- **Description:** Deep breathing involves focusing on slow, deep, and consistent breaths to activate the body's relaxation response, counteracting the stress response.

- **Benefits:** Helps lower heart rate, reduce blood pressure, and promote a state of calm.

- **Practice:** Try the 4-7-8 technique—inhale for 4 seconds, hold for 7 seconds, and exhale for 8 seconds.

Progressive Muscle Relaxation (PMR):

- **Description:** PMR is a technique where you tense each muscle group in the body tightly, but not to the point of strain, and then slowly relax them.

- **Benefits:** Reduces physical tension and mental anxiety, helping to lower stress levels and blood pressure.

- **Practice:** Start from the toes and work your way up to the head, tensing and relaxing each muscle group.

Mindfulness Meditation:

- **Description:** Mindfulness involves paying attention to the present moment without judgment, typically focusing on breath, thoughts, sensations, or emotions.

- **Benefits:** Can decrease stress, anxiety, and symptoms of depression, improving overall well-being and potentially lowering blood pressure.

- **Practice:** Dedicate a few minutes each day to sit quietly and focus on your breath or surroundings.

Physical Activity:

- **Description:** Regular physical activity, including walking, cycling, swimming, or yoga, can significantly reduce stress.

- **Benefits:** Releases endorphins (natural painkillers and mood elevators), improves sleep, and reduces symptoms of mild depression and anxiety.

- **Practice:** Aim for at least 150 minutes of moderate-intensity exercise per week.

Yoga and Tai Chi:

- **Description:** These practices combine physical postures, breathing exercises, meditation, and a philosophical approach to promote physical and mental well-being.

- **Benefits:** Improve flexibility, balance, and strength, while also reducing stress, anxiety, and blood pressure.

- **Practice:** Join a class or find online tutorials to guide you through the basics.

Social Support:

- **Description:** Building and maintaining strong relationships with friends, family, and community.

- **Benefits:** Offers emotional support, reduces feelings of loneliness and isolation, and can help in managing stress.

- **Practice:** Regularly connect with loved ones, whether through social gatherings, phone calls, or digital communication.

Time Management:

- **Description:** Effective time management involves organizing and planning how to divide your time between various activities.

- **Benefits:** Reduces stress by preventing overcommitment and last-minute rushes, allowing for a balanced lifestyle.

- **Practice:** Use planners or digital apps to schedule tasks, set priorities, and delegate when possible.

Hobbies and Leisure Activities:

- **Description:** Engaging in hobbies or activities purely for enjoyment.

- **Benefits:** Provides a break from routine, offers a sense of accomplishment, and reduces stress.

- **Practice:** Dedicate time to pursue interests such as reading, gardening, painting, or playing an instrument.

Conclusion:

Incorporating a variety of stress-reduction techniques into your daily routine can have profound benefits on your mental and physical health, including lowering blood pressure. Experimenting with different methods can help you discover which practices are most effective for you. Remember, managing stress is an ongoing process that requires regular attention and adjustment.

10.3 The Role of Meditation and Relaxation

Meditation and relaxation techniques are powerful tools for managing stress, reducing blood pressure, and enhancing overall well-being. These practices, by promoting a state of calm and relaxation, can counteract the body's stress response, leading to physiological changes that positively impact heart health and hypertension management.

Meditation Techniques:

- **Mindfulness Meditation:** Focuses on being intensely aware of what you're sensing and feeling in the moment, without interpretation or judgment. Practicing mindfulness meditation can reduce stress, anxiety, and blood pressure.

- **Transcendental Meditation:** Involves silently repeating a mantra (a word, sound, or phrase) for 15–20 minutes a day, while sitting comfortably with eyes closed. It's been shown to lower stress levels and blood pressure.

- **Guided Meditation:** Also known as guided imagery or visualization, this method involves forming mental images of places or situations you find relaxing. It's often led by a guide or teacher, making it accessible for beginners.

Relaxation Techniques:

- **Deep Breathing Exercises:** Simple yet effective, deep breathing promotes relaxation and can lower blood pressure by enhancing parasympathetic nervous system activation, which counteracts stress-induced responses.

- **Progressive Muscle Relaxation (PMR):** By tensing and then relaxing each muscle group, PMR helps reduce physical stress and anxiety, which can indirectly lower blood pressure.

- **Autogenic Training:** This technique uses visual imagery and body awareness to reduce stress. You repeat words or suggestions in your mind to relax and reduce muscle tension.

Benefits of Meditation and Relaxation:

- **Reduced Blood Pressure:** Regular practice can lead to reductions in both systolic and diastolic blood pressure by calming the nervous system and reducing stress hormone levels.

- **Improved Stress Management:** Meditation and relaxation techniques improve the ability to cope with stress, reducing the impact of stress on physical health.

- **Enhanced Emotional Well-being:** These practices can improve mood, reduce symptoms of anxiety and depression, and enhance overall well-being.

- **Improved Concentration and Focus:** Regular meditation can increase attention span and focus, making it easier to maintain a healthy lifestyle and manage hypertension.

Implementing Meditation and Relaxation into Your Routine:

- **Consistency is Key:** Even a few minutes of meditation or relaxation each day can yield significant benefits. Establish a regular practice that fits your schedule and lifestyle.

- **Find a Quiet Space:** Choose a quiet, comfortable place where you can relax without interruptions.

- **Use Resources:** Many apps, online videos, and classes offer guided meditations and relaxation exercises for beginners.

- **Be Patient:** Like any skill, meditation and relaxation techniques improve with practice. Be patient with yourself as you learn to quiet your mind and relax your body.

Conclusion:

Incorporating meditation and relaxation practices into your daily routine can be a powerful adjunct to traditional hypertension management strategies. By reducing stress, lowering blood pressure, and improving emotional well-being, these practices contribute to a holistic approach to health and wellness.

10.4 Exercise: 10 MCQs with Answers at the End

Test your understanding of stress management techniques with these multiple-choice questions. Review the answers provided at the end for self-assessment.

1. **Mindfulness meditation focuses on:**

   A. Physical activity to reduce stress

   B. Being aware of the present moment without judgment

   C. Repeating a mantra to enter a state of relaxation

   D. Visualizing peaceful images to calm the mind

2. **Which meditation technique involves silently repeating a mantra?**

    A. Mindfulness Meditation

    B. Transcendental Meditation

    C. Guided Meditation

    D. Autogenic Training

3. **Deep breathing exercises aid in stress management by:**

    A. Increasing heart rate

    B. Reducing blood oxygen levels

    C. Activating the body's relaxation response

    D. Tensing the muscles

4. **Progressive Muscle Relaxation (PMR) is a technique that involves:**

    A. Intense cardio workouts

    B. Tensing and then relaxing each muscle group

    C. Holding breath for extended periods

    D. Rapid eye movement

5. **The primary benefit of meditation and relaxation for hypertension is:**

   A. Immediate lowering of systolic blood pressure by 20 mmHg

   B. Reducing stress and potentially lowering blood pressure

   C. Increasing muscle mass

   D. Enhancing vision clarity

6. **Which of the following is NOT a recognized benefit of regular meditation practice?**

   A. Improved focus and attention

   B. Reduced symptoms of anxiety and depression

   C. Enhanced physical strength

   D. Lowered stress levels

7. **Guided meditation can be particularly helpful for beginners because it:**

   A. Requires special equipment

   B. Involves physical exertion

   C. Is led by a guide or teacher, making it easier to follow

   D. Must be practiced outdoors

8. **Autogenic training focuses on:**

A. Rapid breathing techniques

B. Visual imagery and body awareness to reduce stress

C. Building cardiovascular endurance

D. Increasing flexibility and balance

9. **An effective way to implement meditation into your routine is to:**

A. Practice only when stressed

B. Meditate for several hours each day

C. Establish a regular practice that fits your schedule

D. Wait for perfect conditions before starting

10. **The relaxation response activated by deep breathing exercises counteracts:**

A. The body's immune response

B. The fight or flight response

C. Cognitive function

D. Muscle growth

Answers:

1. B. Being aware of the present moment without judgment

2. B. Transcendental Meditation

3. C. Activating the body's relaxation response

4. B. Tensing and then relaxing each muscle group

5. B. Reducing stress and potentially lowering blood pressure

6. C. Enhanced physical strength

7. C. Is led by a guide or teacher, making it easier to follow

8. B. Visual imagery and body awareness to reduce stress

9. C. Establish a regular practice that fits your schedule

10. B. The fight or flight response

Chapter 11: Monitoring and Self-Care

11.1 Home Blood Pressure Monitoring

Home blood pressure monitoring is an essential component of managing hypertension. It allows individuals to track their blood pressure in the comfort of their own homes, providing valuable information that can help manage and control high blood pressure more effectively. This practice complements clinical measurements and can lead to better long-term management of hypertension.

Benefits of Home Blood Pressure Monitoring:

- **Early Detection:** Helps in the early detection of hypertension or changes in blood pressure patterns.

- **Medication Adjustment:** Assists healthcare providers in adjusting medication doses based on a more comprehensive blood pressure profile.

- **White Coat Hypertension Identification:** Identifies white coat hypertension, where patients have higher blood pressure readings in a clinical setting than at home.

- **Improved Control:** Encourages better blood pressure control through increased awareness and adherence to treatment plans.

- **Self-Empowerment:** Empowers individuals to take an active role in their healthcare.

Choosing a Blood Pressure Monitor:

- **Type:** Automatic, cuff-style, upper-arm monitors are recommended for home use due to their accuracy and ease of use.

- **Validation:** Choose a monitor that has been validated for accuracy and reliability. Organizations like the American Heart Association provide lists of validated devices.

- **Features:** Consider monitors with features that suit your needs, such as memory for storing readings, large display screens, or connectivity to mobile apps.

Proper Use of Home Blood Pressure Monitors:

- **Positioning:** Sit in a comfortable chair with your back supported and feet flat on the floor. Rest your arm on a table at heart level.

- **Timing:** Measure at the same times each day, such as morning and evening, and avoid food, caffeine, tobacco, and exercise for at least 30 minutes before measuring.

- **Consistency:** Use the same arm for measurements, and take two or three readings 1-2 minutes apart to ensure accuracy.

Recording and Sharing Readings:

- Keep a log of your blood pressure readings, noting the date, time, and any relevant circumstances (e.g., after exercise). Many modern monitors can store this information digitally.

- Share your blood pressure log with your healthcare provider during visits to inform adjustments to your treatment plan.

When to Contact a Healthcare Provider:

- If you consistently get readings that are much higher or lower than usual, especially if accompanied by symptoms like headaches, vision problems, or dizziness.

Conclusion:

Home blood pressure monitoring is a vital practice for individuals with hypertension, offering numerous benefits from early detection to enhanced treatment adherence. By selecting an appropriate monitor, using it correctly, and effectively communicating readings with healthcare providers, patients can significantly improve their hypertension management and overall health outcomes.

11.2 Recognizing Changes and When to Act

Recognizing changes in your health, particularly in the context of hypertension, is crucial for timely intervention and preventing complications. By being attentive to your body's signals and understanding when to seek medical advice, you can play an active role in managing your condition. This section outlines key indicators and situations that warrant action or consultation with a healthcare provider.

Blood Pressure Changes:

- **Significant Increase:** Sudden, consistent readings higher than your usual range, especially if they exceed 180/120 mmHg, can indicate a hypertensive crisis. This requires immediate medical attention.

- **Persistent Elevation:** Blood pressure readings consistently above your target range, despite adherence to medication and lifestyle changes, suggest the need for a treatment adjustment.

Symptoms to Watch For:

- **Headaches:** Severe or persistent headaches, especially if not typical for you, can be a sign of elevated blood pressure.

- **Vision Changes:** Blurred vision, double vision, or sudden loss of vision are alarming symptoms that necessitate prompt medical evaluation.

- **Chest Pain or Discomfort:** Any form of chest pain, tightness, or discomfort, particularly if it occurs with physical activity or stress, warrants immediate medical attention.

- **Shortness of Breath:** Difficulty breathing, especially if it occurs at rest or with minimal exertion, can be a sign of heart problems related to hypertension.

- **Dizziness or Fainting Spells:** While these can have many causes, in the context of hypertension, they may signal dangerously high blood pressure or cardiovascular issues.

- **Swelling or Edema:** Unexplained swelling, particularly in the legs, ankles, or feet, can indicate complications from hypertension affecting the heart or kidneys.

Lifestyle and Medication Adherence:

- **Side Effects:** Experiencing adverse effects from medication that impact your quality of life should prompt a discussion with your healthcare provider about possible adjustments.

- **Ineffectiveness:** If lifestyle modifications and medication do not seem to be effectively managing your hypertension, it's important to seek further evaluation and potentially explore alternative treatments.

Regular Check-ups:

- Maintaining regular appointments with your healthcare provider is essential for monitoring hypertension and making timely adjustments to your treatment plan.

Self-Care and Advocacy:

- Be proactive about your health by educating yourself on hypertension and its management, asking questions during medical visits, and advocating for care that addresses your specific needs.

Conclusion:

Recognizing changes in your health and understanding when to act are key components of effective hypertension management. By staying vigilant about symptoms, adhering to treatment plans, and maintaining open communication with healthcare providers, individuals with hypertension can better navigate their condition and minimize the risk of complications.

11.3 Keeping a Health Journal

Maintaining a health journal is a proactive approach to managing hypertension and overall wellness. It involves documenting daily health-related activities, symptoms, blood pressure readings, and any other relevant health information. This practice can enhance self-awareness, improve communication with healthcare providers, and contribute to more personalized and effective hypertension management.

Benefits of Keeping a Health Journal:

- **Tracks Progress and Patterns:** A health journal helps in tracking the effectiveness of medications, lifestyle changes, and their impact on blood pressure over time. Identifying patterns can aid in pinpointing what works best for managing your condition.

- **Enhances Self-Awareness:** Regularly recording your activities, diet, exercise, and how you feel can increase awareness about the factors that influence your blood pressure and overall health.

- **Improves Communication with Healthcare Providers:** A detailed health journal provides your healthcare team with a comprehensive view of your health journey, making it easier to make informed decisions and adjustments to your treatment plan.

- **Motivates and Empowers:** Seeing progress or understanding the challenges in your health journey can motivate you to stick with beneficial habits and feel more in control of your health.

What to Include in a Health Journal:

- **Blood Pressure Readings:** Document your blood pressure readings along with the date and time of day. Note any variations and the possible reasons behind them.

- **Medications:** Keep a record of your medications, dosages, and the timing of your doses. Note any side effects or changes in how you feel.

- **Diet and Nutrition:** Record your daily food and fluid intake, noting meals that are particularly high or low in sodium and potassium, which can affect blood pressure.

- **Physical Activity:** Document your exercise routines, including type, duration, and intensity. Note how you feel during and after exercise.

- **Symptoms and How You Feel:** Record any symptoms you experience, such as headaches, dizziness, or fatigue, and your overall mood or stress levels.

- **Lifestyle Factors:** Include details about your sleep patterns, alcohol consumption, smoking, and any stress management techniques you're using.

- **Questions for Healthcare Providers:** Jot down any questions or concerns you want to discuss during your next appointment.

Tips for Maintaining a Health Journal:

- **Consistency:** Try to make entries regularly, whether daily or several times a week, to ensure your journal accurately reflects your health over time.

- **Accessibility:** Keep your journal in a format that's easy for you to maintain, whether it's a traditional notebook, a digital document, or a specialized app.

- **Review and Reflect:** Periodically review your journal to assess progress, identify areas for improvement, and prepare for discussions with your healthcare team.

Conclusion:

A health journal is a valuable tool in the management of hypertension, offering insights into the relationship between lifestyle choices, medication, and blood pressure control. By diligently recording and reviewing health-related information, individuals can play an active role in their healthcare, leading to more tailored treatment strategies and improved outcomes.

11.4 Exercise: 10 MCQs with Answers at the End

Assess your understanding of monitoring and self-care for hypertension with these multiple-choice questions. Review the answers at the end to gauge your comprehension.

1. **The primary purpose of home blood pressure monitoring is to:**

   A. Replace regular doctor visits

   B. Identify patterns and changes in blood pressure

   C. Test the accuracy of professional medical equipment

   D. Provide data for academic research

2. **A sudden and consistent rise in blood pressure readings above normal might indicate:**

   A. The need for immediate relaxation

   B. An error in measurement technique

   C. The necessity for a medication adjustment

   D. That exercise is working effectively

3. **Key benefits of maintaining a health journal include all except:**

A. Enhanced medication adherence

B. Reduced need for hypertension medication

C. Improved communication with healthcare providers

D. Better awareness of health patterns

4. **Which symptom should prompt immediate consultation with a healthcare provider when monitoring hypertension?**

A. Temporary muscle soreness after exercise

B. Severe or persistent headaches

C. Occasional fatigue

D. Mild indigestion

5. **Effective stress management techniques for hypertension might include:**

A. Increasing caffeine intake

B. Practicing deep breathing exercises

C. Reducing the amount of sleep

D. Ignoring stressors

6. **When documenting diet in a health journal, it's important to note:**

A. Only the caloric content of meals

B. Every single ingredient in every dish

C. High or low sodium and potassium foods

D. The brand names of all consumed foods

7. **A health journal helps in managing hypertension by:**

A. Providing entertainment through journaling

B. Tracking progress and identifying triggers

C. Eliminating the need for hypertension medication

D. Guaranteeing a reduction in blood pressure

8. **Regular physical activity benefits those with hypertension by:**

A. Increasing long-term dependence on medications

B. Lowering heart rate and improving blood vessel flexibility

C. Exclusively reducing systolic blood pressure

D. Eliminating the need for dietary management

9. **Symptoms of overexertion during exercise include:**

A. Gradual heart rate increase during activity

B. Dizziness and chest pain

C. Feeling energized

D. Slow breathing

10. The practice of progressive muscle relaxation involves:

A. Holding breath for extended periods

B. Tensing and then relaxing each muscle group

C. Rapid, shallow breathing

D. High-intensity interval training

Answers:

1. **B. Identify patterns and changes in blood pressure**

2. **C. The necessity for a medication adjustment**

3. **B. Reduced need for hypertension medication**

4. **B. Severe or persistent headaches**

5. **B. Practicing deep breathing exercises**

6. **C. High or low sodium and potassium foods**

7. **B. Tracking progress and identifying triggers**

8. **B. Lowering heart rate and improving blood vessel flexibility**

9. **B. Dizziness and chest pain**

10. **B. Tensing and then relaxing each muscle group**

Chapter 12: The Role of Healthcare Professionals

12.1 Choosing the Right Doctor

For individuals managing hypertension, selecting the right healthcare professional is crucial for receiving effective care and support. A healthcare provider who understands your unique health needs, communicates clearly, and collaborates with you in managing your condition can significantly impact your health outcomes. Here's how to make an informed choice.

Types of Healthcare Providers for Hypertension Management:

- **Primary Care Physicians (PCPs):** Often the first point of contact, PCPs can diagnose and treat hypertension, coordinate care, and refer patients to specialists as needed.

- **Cardiologists:** Specialists in heart health who can provide advanced care for patients with severe hypertension or related cardiovascular conditions.

- **Nephrologists:** Specialists in kidney health, essential for patients where hypertension is linked to or affecting renal function.

- **Endocrinologists:** For patients whose hypertension may be related to hormonal issues, such as thyroid problems or adrenal disorders.

Factors to Consider When Choosing a Doctor:

- **Credentials and Experience:** Look for board certification in their specialty, indicating they have the necessary training, skills, and experience to provide healthcare in their field.

- **Communication Style:** Choose a doctor who listens to your concerns, explains things clearly, and involves you in decision-making processes.

- **Accessibility:** Consider the location of their office, office hours, and whether they offer telehealth services for convenience.

- **Insurance Coverage:** Ensure the doctor is within your health insurance network to avoid unexpected medical costs.

- **Patient Reviews and Recommendations:** Look for feedback from other patients about their experiences with the doctor or ask for recommendations from friends, family, or other healthcare professionals.

Building a Relationship with Your Healthcare Provider:

- **Be Open and Honest:** Share your medical history, lifestyle habits, and any concerns or symptoms you're experiencing.

- **Prepare for Appointments:** Bring a list of your current medications, recent blood pressure readings, questions you have, and any notes from your health journal.

- **Follow Through on Recommendations:** Adhere to prescribed treatment plans, including medication, lifestyle changes, and follow-up appointments.

Changing Doctors:

- If you feel your healthcare needs are not being met or if there are communication issues, it's acceptable to look for another doctor. Your health and comfort with your care provider are paramount.

Conclusion:

Choosing the right healthcare professional is a key step in managing hypertension effectively. By considering factors such as credentials, communication style, accessibility, and insurance coverage, you can select a provider who best fits your health needs and preferences. A strong, collaborative relationship with your healthcare provider can lead to better management of hypertension and improved overall health.

12.2 Working with a Healthcare Team

Effective management of hypertension often requires a multidisciplinary approach, involving various healthcare professionals who contribute their expertise to your overall care plan. Collaborating closely with a healthcare team can help address the complexities of hypertension, ensuring that all aspects of your health are considered. This integrated approach promotes comprehensive care, tailored to your unique needs and health goals.

Members of a Healthcare Team for Hypertension Management:

- **Primary Care Physicians (PCPs):** Serve as the central figure in managing your overall health, including diagnosing hypertension, prescribing medications, and making referrals to specialists.

- **Cardiologists:** Specialists who manage complex cardiovascular issues related to hypertension, such as heart disease or heart failure.

- **Nephrologists:** Focus on kidney health, especially relevant if hypertension has affected kidney function or if kidney issues are contributing to high blood pressure.

- **Dietitians or Nutritionists:** Provide guidance on dietary changes that can help control blood pressure, such as reducing sodium intake and adopting the DASH diet.

- **Pharmacists:** Offer advice on medication management, including how to take medications correctly, side effects, and interactions with other drugs or supplements.

- **Nurses and Nurse Practitioners:** Often the first point of contact in clinical settings, they provide education, monitor your condition, and help manage your care plan.

- **Mental Health Professionals:** Address the psychological aspects of living with a chronic condition like hypertension, including stress, anxiety, and depression.

- **Physical Therapists or Exercise Physiologists:** Advise on safe and effective physical activities and exercises that can help lower blood pressure and improve cardiovascular health.

Benefits of Working with a Healthcare Team:

- **Comprehensive Care:** A team approach ensures that all factors contributing to hypertension, including lifestyle, diet, medication, and coexisting conditions, are addressed.

- **Personalized Treatment:** Collaborating with specialists allows for treatment plans to be customized to your specific health needs and goals.

- **Consistent Monitoring:** Regular check-ups with your healthcare team help track progress, make necessary adjustments to treatment, and promptly address any emerging health issues.

- **Support and Education:** The diverse expertise within the team provides a wealth of knowledge, offering education on managing hypertension and support for making lifestyle changes.

Tips for Effective Collaboration with Your Healthcare Team:

- **Communicate Openly:** Share your health concerns, experiences, and preferences with your team. Honest communication is key to effective care.

- **Stay Informed:** Educate yourself about hypertension and its management to engage in informed discussions with your healthcare providers.

- **Follow Through:** Adhere to the treatment plan agreed upon with your team, including taking medications as prescribed, making lifestyle changes, and attending follow-up appointments.

- **Ask Questions:** Don't hesitate to ask for clarification or further information about any aspect of your care. Understanding your treatment plan is crucial for successful management.

Conclusion:

Managing hypertension effectively often requires the expertise and support of a multidisciplinary healthcare team. By actively engaging with and leveraging the diverse skills of your healthcare providers, you can achieve better control over your blood pressure, reduce the risk of complications, and improve your overall quality of life.

12.3 Questions to Ask Your Doctor

Effective communication with your healthcare provider is crucial in managing hypertension. Preparing questions in advance can help you make the most of your appointments and ensure that you understand your condition, treatment options, and what you can do to manage your blood pressure effectively. Here are some key questions to consider asking your doctor during your next visit:

1. **What is my blood pressure reading, and what do these numbers mean?**

   - Understanding your readings can help you grasp the severity of your hypertension and the risks associated with your specific levels.

2. **What is my target blood pressure, and how can I achieve it?**

- Knowing your target can help you monitor your progress and adjust your management strategies as needed.

3. What are the potential causes or contributing factors to my hypertension?

- Identifying underlying causes can aid in tailoring your treatment plan.

4. What lifestyle changes do you recommend to help manage my blood pressure?

- Lifestyle modifications, such as diet and exercise, play a crucial role in managing hypertension.

5. How does my current medication work, and what are the possible side effects?

- Understanding how your medications affect your body can help you recognize and manage side effects.

6. Do I need to monitor my blood pressure at home, and if so, how often?

- Home monitoring can provide valuable insights into your blood pressure patterns and the effectiveness of your treatment.

7. Are there any dietary restrictions I should follow, such as limiting sodium or alcohol?

- Dietary adjustments can significantly impact blood pressure control.

8. Should I be limiting or avoiding any specific activities or exercises?

- Certain activities may not be suitable depending on your condition and fitness level.

9. How does my hypertension affect my risk for other health conditions, such as heart disease or kidney damage?

- Hypertension can increase the risk of various complications, making it important to understand your overall health risks.

10. What should I do if I experience side effects from my medication or if my blood pressure readings change significantly?

- Knowing how to respond to these situations can help you manage your condition more effectively.

11. Are there any resources or support groups you recommend for patients with hypertension?

- Additional resources can provide support, education, and motivation to manage your condition.

12. How often should I schedule follow-up appointments to monitor my hypertension?

- Regular check-ups allow for adjustments to your treatment plan and ensure that your blood pressure is adequately controlled.

Preparing and asking these questions can help you gain a better understanding of your hypertension and how to manage it effectively. It also strengthens the partnership between you and your healthcare provider, fostering a collaborative approach to your health care.

12.4 Exercise: 10 MCQs with Answers at the End

Test your knowledge on the role of healthcare professionals in hypertension management with these multiple-choice questions. Review the answers provided at the end to assess your understanding.

1. **Who is typically the central figure in managing an individual's hypertension?**

   A. Cardiologist

   B. Primary Care Physician (PCP)

   C. Nephrologist

   D. Dietitian

2. **What is the primary role of a cardiologist in hypertension management?**

   A. Provide dietary advice

   B. Manage complex cardiovascular issues related to hypertension

   C. Prescribe all necessary medications

   D. Offer psychological support

3. **Why might someone with hypertension be referred to a nephrologist?**

   A. If they need surgery

   B. If their hypertension is linked to kidney function

   C. For routine blood pressure checks

   D. To learn stress management techniques

4. **A dietitian can help a patient with hypertension by:**

   A. Performing heart surgery

   B. Prescribing blood pressure medication

   C. Providing guidance on dietary changes to control blood pressure

   D. Diagnosing the type of hypertension

5. **Which healthcare professional might offer advice on medication management, including side effects and interactions?**

A. Pharmacist

B. Physical Therapist

C. Mental Health Professional

D. Exercise Physiologist

6. **What is one benefit of keeping a health journal for hypertension management?**

A. It eliminates the need for medication

B. It can improve communication with healthcare providers

C. It guarantees a cure for hypertension

D. It allows for self-prescription of medications

7. **Which of the following is NOT a common reason for changing doctors?**

A. Preference for a doctor of a specific gender

B. Disagreements over the importance of blood pressure control

C. Communication issues

D. Seeking a specialist for a related health condition

8. Regular physical activity is recommended for individuals with hypertension because it:

A. Allows for higher sodium intake

B. Reduces the need for sleep

C. Lowers heart rate and improves blood vessel flexibility

D. Increases dependence on medication

9. Effective stress management for someone with hypertension might include:

A. Increasing caffeine consumption

B. Practicing mindfulness meditation

C. Ignoring symptoms of stress

D. Limiting hours of sleep

10. When preparing for a doctor's appointment, it's helpful to:

A. Bring a list of current medications and recent blood pressure readings

B. Wait for the doctor to ask all the questions

C. Assume the doctor remembers all your medical history

D. Avoid mentioning any new symptoms

Answers:

1. **B. Primary Care Physician (PCP)**

2. **B. Manage complex cardiovascular issues related to hypertension**

3. **B. If their hypertension is linked to kidney function**

4. **C. Providing guidance on dietary changes to control blood pressure**

5. **A. Pharmacist**

6. **B. It can improve communication with healthcare providers**

7. **A. Preference for a doctor of a specific gender**

8. **C. Lowers heart rate and improves blood vessel flexibility**

9. **B. Practicing mindfulness meditation**

10. **A. Bring a list of current medications and recent blood pressure readings**

Chapter 13: Future Directions in Hypertension Care

13.1 Emerging Treatments and Therapies

The field of hypertension care is continually evolving, with research and technological advancements leading to new and innovative treatments. These emerging therapies aim to provide more effective, personalized, and less invasive options for managing high blood pressure. Here's a glimpse into some of the promising developments in hypertension care.

Renal Denervation (RDN):

- **Overview:** A minimally invasive procedure that uses radiofrequency ablation or ultrasound to disrupt the renal nerves, which play a role in blood pressure regulation. Initial studies suggest that RDN can significantly reduce blood pressure in patients with resistant hypertension, who do not respond adequately to medication.

- **Current Status:** Ongoing clinical trials are evaluating the long-term efficacy and safety of RDN. While not yet widely available, early results are promising.

Baroreflex Activation Therapy (BAT):

- **Overview:** BAT involves the implantation of a device that electrically stimulates the baroreceptors in the carotid artery, enhancing the body's natural blood pressure regulation mechanisms. It's designed for patients with drug-resistant hypertension.

- **Current Status:** Currently under investigation, with some clinical trials showing positive outcomes in lowering blood pressure and improving patient quality of life.

Polygenic Risk Scoring:

- **Overview:** This approach uses genetic testing to assess an individual's risk of developing hypertension based on the presence of multiple genetic markers. It aims to enable early intervention and personalized treatment strategies based on genetic predisposition.

- **Current Status:** Research in this area is expanding, with the potential to integrate genetic risk scoring into routine clinical practice for targeted prevention and treatment.

Wearable Technology for Continuous Blood Pressure Monitoring:

- **Overview:** Advances in wearable technology are leading to the development of devices capable of continuous, non-invasive blood pressure monitoring. These devices could provide real-time data, allowing for more dynamic management of hypertension.

- **Current Status:** While several devices are in development or early deployment stages, accuracy and reliability continue to be areas of focus for research and improvement.

Novel Medications and Drug Combinations:

- **Overview:** Ongoing research into the pathways involved in hypertension is leading to the development of new pharmacological treatments. These include drugs targeting different mechanisms of action, as well as optimized combinations of existing medications to improve efficacy and reduce side effects.

- **Current Status:** Several new medications and combinations are in various stages of clinical trials, with some showing promising results in managing hypertension more effectively and safely.

Conclusion:

The future of hypertension care is bright, with numerous emerging treatments and therapies on the horizon. These advancements promise to enhance our ability to manage hypertension more effectively, reduce the incidence of cardiovascular complications, and improve the quality of life for individuals with high blood pressure. As these new technologies and treatments undergo further study and development, they hold the potential to significantly impact the landscape of hypertension management.

13.2 Technological Advances in Monitoring

The landscape of hypertension monitoring is undergoing significant transformation, thanks to technological advancements. These innovations aim to improve the accuracy, convenience, and effectiveness of blood pressure monitoring, making it easier for patients and healthcare providers to track and manage hypertension in real-time. Let's explore some of the notable technological advances in this area.

Wearable Blood Pressure Monitors:

- **Overview:** Wearable devices, such as smartwatches and fitness bands, are being developed to offer continuous, non-invasive blood pressure monitoring throughout the day. These devices use various technologies, including optical sensors and tonometry, to measure blood pressure without the need for a traditional cuff.

- **Benefits:** Continuous monitoring can provide a more comprehensive picture of an individual's blood pressure patterns, including variations related to activity, sleep, and stress, which can inform better treatment decisions.

Smartphone Applications:

- **Overview:** Smartphone apps designed for hypertension management can track blood pressure readings, medication schedules, and lifestyle factors. Some apps also offer educational content, reminders, and personalized feedback.

- **Benefits:** These applications enhance patient engagement and adherence to treatment plans by making it easier to record and visualize data, set reminders for medications, and understand the impact of lifestyle choices on blood pressure.

Remote Patient Monitoring (RPM) Systems:

- **Overview:** RPM systems allow healthcare providers to monitor patients' blood pressure and other health metrics remotely. Patients use connected devices at home to take readings, which are then automatically transmitted to healthcare providers for review.

- **Benefits:** RPM can improve access to care, especially for patients in remote areas or with mobility issues, and facilitate timely interventions based on real-time data.

Advanced Analytical Tools:

- **Overview:** The integration of artificial intelligence (AI) and machine learning algorithms with blood pressure monitoring technologies is enabling the development of advanced analytical tools. These tools can predict blood pressure trends, identify risk factors, and personalize treatment recommendations.

- **Benefits:** AI-enhanced analytics can lead to more accurate risk assessment, early detection of potential complications, and tailored treatment strategies, improving overall outcomes.

Telehealth and Virtual Consultations:

- **Overview:** The rise of telehealth services, including virtual consultations with healthcare providers, complements technological advances in blood pressure monitoring by facilitating discussions about treatment adjustments, lifestyle recommendations, and medication management based on remotely collected data.

- **Benefits:** Virtual care options increase the convenience and frequency of patient-provider interactions, enhancing the management of hypertension and patient satisfaction.

Conclusion:

Technological advances in monitoring are revolutionizing the management of hypertension, offering new opportunities for early detection, continuous monitoring, and personalized care. As these technologies continue to evolve and gain validation, they promise to integrate seamlessly into hypertension care, empowering patients and providers with more precise, real-time data to guide treatment decisions and improve health outcomes.

13.3 The Role of Personalized Medicine

Personalized medicine, also known as precision medicine, represents a shift from a one-size-fits-all approach to healthcare towards tailored strategies based on an individual's genetic makeup, lifestyle, and environmental factors. In the context of hypertension, personalized medicine offers the promise of more effective management by identifying the most suitable treatments and preventative measures for each individual. This approach could significantly enhance patient outcomes, particularly for those with resistant or complicated forms of hypertension.

Genetic Testing and Hypertension:

- **Overview:** Genetic testing can identify specific genetic variants that contribute to the risk of developing hypertension. This knowledge allows healthcare providers to predict the likelihood of hypertension development, understand its potential severity, and tailor interventions accordingly.

- **Benefits:** Early intervention in individuals identified as high-risk can prevent the onset of hypertension or mitigate its impact. Moreover, understanding genetic contributions can guide the selection of medications that are more likely to be effective for specific individuals.

Pharmacogenomics:

- **Overview:** Pharmacogenomics examines how genes affect an individual's response to drugs. This field is particularly relevant for hypertension management, where there can be significant variability in how patients respond to antihypertensive medications.

- **Benefits:** By considering genetic factors, healthcare providers can choose medications that are more likely to be effective and have fewer side effects for the individual, improving treatment adherence and outcomes.

Lifestyle and Environmental Factors:

- **Overview:** Personalized medicine also considers an individual's lifestyle and environmental factors, such as diet, physical activity, stress levels, and exposure to pollutants, which can influence blood pressure.

- **Benefits:** Tailored lifestyle recommendations can complement pharmacological treatments, providing a holistic approach to hypertension management that is specifically adapted to each individual's circumstances.

Digital Health and Data Analytics:

- **Overview:** The integration of digital health tools, such as wearable devices and mobile health apps, with data analytics allows for continuous monitoring and collection of health-related data. Analyzing this data can uncover patterns and predict outcomes, guiding personalized interventions.

- **Benefits:** Real-time monitoring and personalized feedback can help individuals make informed decisions about their health, adjust their lifestyle, and manage their hypertension more effectively.

Challenges and Considerations:

- **Ethical and Privacy Concerns:** The use of genetic information and continuous health monitoring raises ethical and privacy concerns that need to be addressed through strict data protection measures.

- **Accessibility and Cost:** Ensuring that personalized medicine approaches are accessible to all patients, regardless of socioeconomic status, is crucial for equitable healthcare delivery.

Conclusion:

The role of personalized medicine in hypertension care is expanding, offering new avenues for diagnosing, treating, and preventing this common and complex condition. By harnessing genetic insights, lifestyle data, and advanced analytics, personalized medicine can provide tailored and effective hypertension management strategies. As research advances and these practices become more integrated into clinical care, they hold the potential to significantly improve outcomes for individuals with hypertension.

13.4 Exercise: 10 MCQs with Answers at the End

Test your understanding of the future directions in hypertension care with these multiple-choice questions. Review the answers provided at the end for self-assessment.

1. **Renal Denervation (RDN) is a treatment for hypertension that involves:**

   A. Dietary changes

   B. Genetic modification

   C. Disrupting renal nerves

D. Increasing kidney filtration

2. Baroreflex Activation Therapy (BAT) is designed for patients with:

A. Mild hypertension

B. Drug-resistant hypertension

C. Kidney disease

D. Genetic predispositions to hypertension

3. Polygenic risk scoring in hypertension aims to:

A. Replace traditional blood pressure monitoring

B. Predict hypertension based on genetic markers

C. Increase the effectiveness of antihypertensive drugs

D. Identify suitable dietary interventions

4. Wearable technology for blood pressure monitoring offers the benefit of:

A. Eliminating the need for medication

B. Providing continuous, non-invasive monitoring

C. Serving as a replacement for healthcare provider visits

D. Guaranteeing the reduction of blood pressure

5. **Pharmacogenomics in hypertension care helps in:**

    A. Designing new exercise programs

    B. Choosing medications based on genetic makeup

    C. Predicting the future development of hypertension

    D. Eliminating the need for lifestyle changes

6. **The primary challenge in implementing personalized medicine in hypertension care includes:**

    A. Lack of evidence for its effectiveness

    B. Ethical and privacy concerns

    C. The need for frequent blood pressure readings

    D. Patients' reluctance to use digital health tools

7. **Emerging treatments like RDN and BAT are particularly aimed at patients with:**

    A. Early-stage hypertension

    B. Hypertension caused by stress

    C. Resistant or uncontrolled hypertension

    D. Hypertension without any genetic basis

8. Continuous monitoring of blood pressure through wearable technology can help:

A. Cure hypertension

B. Identify blood pressure patterns and triggers

C. Serve as the sole method for diagnosing hypertension

D. Replace all other forms of blood pressure management

9. In the context of hypertension, personalized medicine focuses on:

A. Treating all patients with the same methodology

B. Tailoring treatment based on genetic, lifestyle, and environmental factors

C. Focusing solely on genetic factors

D. Disregarding traditional blood pressure management techniques

10. Advancements in data analytics and artificial intelligence in hypertension care aim to:

A. Completely automate patient care without human oversight

B. Predict blood pressure trends and personalize treatment recommendations

C. Reduce the importance of lifestyle modifications in managing hypertension

D. Focus exclusively on developing new surgical techniques

Answers:

1. **C. Disrupting renal nerves**

2. **B. Drug-resistant hypertension**

3. **B. Predict hypertension based on genetic markers**

4. **B. Providing continuous, non-invasive monitoring**

5. **B. Choosing medications based on genetic makeup**

6. **B. Ethical and privacy concerns**

7. **C. Resistant or uncontrolled hypertension**

8. **B. Identify blood pressure patterns and triggers**

9. **B. Tailoring treatment based on genetic, lifestyle, and environmental factors**

10. **B. Predict blood pressure trends and personalize treatment recommendations**

Chapter 14: Lifestyle Changes for Prevention

14.1 The Power of Prevention

Preventing hypertension is crucial in reducing the risk of heart disease, stroke, and other serious health complications. Lifestyle changes play a foundational role in preventing high blood pressure, offering a powerful means to not only avoid the onset of hypertension but also improve overall health and quality of life. This approach is centered on adopting healthy habits that support heart health and maintain blood pressure within a normal range.

Key Lifestyle Changes for Hypertension Prevention:

Healthy Diet:

- Adopting a diet rich in fruits, vegetables, whole grains, and lean proteins can significantly impact blood pressure. The DASH (Dietary Approaches to Stop Hypertension) diet is specifically designed to prevent and lower high blood pressure.

- Reducing sodium intake is crucial, as excessive sodium can increase blood pressure. Aim for less than 2,300 mg of sodium per day, moving toward an ideal limit of no more than 1,500 mg for most adults.

- Limiting alcohol consumption and avoiding foods high in saturated fats and added sugars also contribute to maintaining healthy blood pressure levels.

Regular Physical Activity:

- Engaging in regular physical activity, such as brisk walking, cycling, swimming, or jogging, can help prevent hypertension and promote heart health. The American Heart Association recommends at least 150 minutes of moderate-intensity aerobic activity or 75 minutes of vigorous aerobic activity per week, or a combination of both.

- Strength training exercises at least two days a week complement aerobic activities and contribute to overall cardiovascular health.

Weight Management:

- Maintaining a healthy weight is key to preventing high blood pressure. Losing even a small amount of weight if you're overweight or obese can have a significant impact on lowering blood pressure.

- Body mass index (BMI) and waist circumference are useful measures to assess weight status and risk associated with obesity.

Stress Management:

- Chronic stress can contribute to elevated blood pressure. Techniques such as mindfulness, deep breathing exercises, yoga, and spending time on hobbies can help manage stress effectively.

- Developing healthy coping strategies for dealing with life's challenges can prevent stress from negatively impacting blood pressure.

Avoidance of Tobacco Use:

- Smoking and tobacco use can raise blood pressure and increase the risk of heart disease. Quitting smoking can improve heart health and lower the risk of developing hypertension.

Regular Health Screenings:

- Regular blood pressure screenings can help detect prehypertension or early stages of hypertension, allowing for timely intervention with lifestyle changes or medication if necessary.

Conclusion:

The power of prevention lies in the adoption of healthy lifestyle changes. By focusing on a nutritious diet, regular physical activity, weight management, stress reduction, and avoiding harmful substances like tobacco, individuals can significantly reduce their risk of developing hypertension. These changes not only prevent high blood pressure but also contribute to a healthier, more vibrant life.

14.2 Building Healthy Habits

Building healthy habits is essential for preventing hypertension and maintaining overall well-being. It involves making conscious decisions to engage in activities that promote health while avoiding those that pose risks. Establishing these habits can be challenging, but with patience, persistence, and a strategic approach, it's achievable. Here are steps and strategies to build healthy habits that can help prevent hypertension and enhance your quality of life.

Start Small:

- Focus on making small changes first, such as adding an extra serving of vegetables to your meals or taking a short walk daily. Small successes can build confidence and motivation to take on larger challenges.

Set Clear, Achievable Goals:

- Define specific, measurable, attainable, relevant, and time-bound (SMART) goals. For example, "I will walk for 30 minutes at a moderate pace five days a week" is clearer and more achievable than a vague intention to "exercise more."

Understand Your Motivations:

- Identify why you want to build these habits. Understanding the personal benefits, whether it's improving health, feeling better, or setting a good example for family members, can keep you motivated.

Create a Supportive Environment:

- Make your environment conducive to change. This can mean stocking your kitchen with healthy food options, finding a workout buddy, or removing temptations that lead to unhealthy behaviors.

Establish Routine and Consistency:

- Incorporate new habits into your daily routine to make them a part of your lifestyle. Consistency reinforces habits, making them more automatic over time.

Track Your Progress:

- Keep a journal or use apps to track your progress towards your goals. Seeing improvements, whether in physical activity levels, dietary choices, or weight management, can provide encouragement.

Reward Yourself:

- Celebrate milestones and rewards yourself with non-food-related rewards, such as a new book, a day out, or time for a favorite hobby.

Be Prepared for Setbacks:

- Understand that setbacks are part of the process. Instead of being discouraged, learn from them and adjust your strategies as needed.

Seek Professional Guidance:

- Consult with healthcare providers, nutritionists, or fitness experts to get personalized advice tailored to your health status and goals.

Stay Informed:

- Keep up-to-date with the latest health information and recommendations. Knowledge is empowering and can inspire you to maintain your healthy habits.

Incorporate Mindfulness:

- Practice mindfulness to stay present and make conscious choices about your health. Being mindful can help you recognize triggers for unhealthy behaviors and respond in healthier ways.

Conclusion:

Building healthy habits is a journey that requires time, effort, and commitment. By starting small, setting clear goals, and staying consistent, you can develop a lifestyle that supports the prevention of hypertension and promotes overall health and well-being. Remember, the key to success is persistence and a positive outlook, even in the face of challenges.

14.3 Community and Support Networks

The role of community and support networks in promoting healthy habits and preventing hypertension cannot be overstated. Having a support system can significantly enhance motivation, accountability, and persistence in adopting and maintaining lifestyle changes crucial for blood pressure management. Here's how engaging with community and support networks can make a difference and ways to find or build these networks.

Benefits of Community and Support Networks:

- **Shared Experiences:** Connecting with others facing similar health challenges provides a sense of belonging and understanding. Shared experiences can offer practical advice, emotional support, and motivation.

- **Accountability:** Being part of a group or having a health buddy increases accountability. It's easier to stick with a fitness routine, dietary changes, or medication schedules when you know someone else is supporting you and perhaps even participating with you.

- **Access to Resources and Information:** Support groups and community networks often provide valuable resources and information about managing hypertension, including tips on diet, exercise, stress reduction, and medication adherence.

- **Emotional Support:** Knowing you're not alone in your health journey can provide significant emotional relief. Support networks offer a safe space to express concerns, celebrate successes, and navigate setbacks.

Finding or Building a Support Network:

- **Local Support Groups:** Many communities have support groups for individuals with hypertension or general heart health. Hospitals, clinics, and community centers often host these groups.

- **Online Forums and Social Media:** Online platforms can connect you with individuals worldwide. Websites, forums, and social media groups focused on hypertension and cardiovascular health are valuable resources.

- **Fitness Clubs or Classes:** Joining a fitness club, gym, or class (like yoga or walking clubs) can provide a community with similar health goals. Group activities can make exercise more enjoyable and consistent.

- **Nutritional Workshops and Cooking Classes:** Participating in workshops focused on healthy eating can introduce you to people striving for similar dietary changes. It's also a great way to learn new skills and recipes.

- **Family and Friends:** Sometimes, your existing network can be your best support. Engaging family and friends in your health goals can provide a built-in support system for encouragement and accountability.

- **Healthcare Professionals:** Doctors, nurses, dietitians, and fitness trainers can offer professional support, guiding you through the complexities of managing hypertension.

Maximizing the Benefits of Your Support Network:

- **Be Active:** Engage actively in your community or support group by attending meetings, participating in discussions, and sharing your experiences.

- **Set Collective Goals:** Working towards common goals can strengthen your commitment and provide a sense of collective achievement.

- **Respect Privacy:** While sharing can be beneficial, it's important to respect the privacy of others, just as you would want your privacy respected.

- **Offer Support:** Remember that support networks are reciprocal. Offering encouragement and support to others can strengthen your sense of purpose and connection.

Conclusion:

Community and support networks play a vital role in preventing hypertension and promoting a healthy lifestyle. By finding or building a support system, you can enhance your ability to adopt and maintain the changes necessary for managing blood pressure and improving your overall health and well-being.

14.4 Exercise: 10 MCQs with Answers at the End

Evaluate your understanding of lifestyle changes for hypertension prevention with these multiple-choice questions. Check your answers at the end for self-assessment.

1. **The DASH diet specifically targets:**

   A. Weight loss

   B. High blood sugar

   C. High blood pressure

   D. High cholesterol

2. **Regular physical activity reduces hypertension risk by:**

   A. Decreasing lung capacity

   B. Increasing blood volume

   C. Lowering heart rate and improving blood vessel flexibility

   D. Increasing sodium retention

3. **For effective hypertension prevention, adults should aim for a minimum of:**

   A. 75 minutes of vigorous aerobic activity per week

   B. 150 minutes of moderate-intensity aerobic activity per week

   C. 200 minutes of light physical activity per week

   D. A and B are correct

4. **Which of the following is not a recommended dietary change for hypertension prevention?**

A. Increasing potassium intake

B. Reducing sodium intake

C. Consuming more saturated fats

D. Limiting alcohol consumption

5. **Stress management techniques beneficial for preventing hypertension include:**

A. Deep breathing exercises

B. Increasing caffeine intake

C. Ignoring stressors

D. Avoiding physical activity

6. **Maintaining a healthy weight is important because obesity:**

A. Decreases blood volume

B. Reduces heart rate

C. Increases the risk of developing hypertension

D. Lowers cholesterol levels

7. **Which lifestyle habit is known to directly increase blood pressure and should be avoided?**

A. Tobacco use

B. Regular exercise

C. Sleeping 7-8 hours per night

D. Eating whole grains

8. **Community support in hypertension prevention can provide:**

A. A platform for competitive sports

B. Financial assistance for medications

C. Emotional support and shared experiences

D. A guaranteed cure for hypertension

9. **The role of a support network in managing hypertension includes:**

A. Prescribing medications

B. Providing accountability and motivation

C. Performing surgical interventions

D. Offering legal advice

10. **Effective stress management has been shown to impact blood pressure by:**

A. Increasing stress hormone levels

B. Decreasing stress hormone levels and promoting relaxation

C. Increasing blood glucose levels

D. Decreasing immune system function

Answers:

1. **C. High blood pressure**

2. **C. Lowering heart rate and improving blood vessel flexibility**

3. **D. A and B are correct**

4. **C. Consuming more saturated fats**

5. **A. Deep breathing exercises**

6. **C. Increases the risk of developing hypertension**

7. **A. Tobacco use**

8. **C. Emotional support and shared experiences**

9. **B. Providing accountability and motivation**

10. **B. Decreasing stress hormone levels and promoting relaxation**

Chapter 15: Living with Hypertension

15.1 Long-Term Management Strategies

Living with hypertension requires a comprehensive and sustained approach to ensure long-term health and prevent complications. Effective management involves a combination of medication, lifestyle adjustments, regular monitoring, and communication with healthcare professionals. Here are key strategies for long-term management of hypertension.

Medication Adherence:

- **Consistency:** Taking prescribed medication consistently as directed by a healthcare provider is crucial. Missed doses can lead to fluctuations in blood pressure.

- **Communication:** Discuss any side effects or concerns with medications with your healthcare provider. There may be alternatives or adjustments that can improve tolerability and effectiveness.

Lifestyle Modifications:

- **Diet:** Maintain a heart-healthy diet low in sodium and rich in fruits, vegetables, whole grains, and lean proteins. The DASH diet is specifically designed to help manage blood pressure.

- **Physical Activity:** Incorporate regular physical activity into your routine, aiming for at least 150 minutes of moderate-intensity aerobic exercise per week.

- **Weight Management:** Strive to maintain a healthy weight. Even a small amount of weight loss can have a significant impact on blood pressure control.

- **Limit Alcohol and Avoid Tobacco:** Limiting alcohol intake and avoiding tobacco use can lower blood pressure and reduce the risk of heart disease.

Regular Monitoring and Check-ups:

- **Home Monitoring:** Regularly monitor your blood pressure at home to track your progress and identify any changes that may require attention.

- **Healthcare Visits:** Keep up with regular healthcare appointments to monitor your condition, adjust treatment plans, and address any health concerns.

Stress Management:

- **Techniques:** Employ stress reduction techniques such as deep breathing, meditation, yoga, or hobbies that you enjoy. Managing stress can help control blood pressure.

- **Support:** Seek support from friends, family, or support groups. Sharing your experiences and challenges can provide emotional relief and valuable advice.

Education and Empowerment:

- **Stay Informed:** Educate yourself about hypertension, its risks, and the latest management strategies. Understanding your condition empowers you to make informed decisions about your care.

- **Advocate for Yourself:** Be proactive in your healthcare. Ask questions, seek second opinions if necessary, and ensure you fully understand and agree with your treatment plan.

Dealing with Complications:

- Be aware of the potential complications associated with hypertension, such as heart disease, stroke, and kidney damage. Promptly addressing symptoms or changes in your condition can prevent or mitigate these complications.

Conclusion:

Long-term management of hypertension involves a multifaceted approach that includes medication adherence, lifestyle changes, regular monitoring, stress management, and proactive healthcare engagement. By taking an active role in managing your condition, you can live a healthy and fulfilling life despite hypertension. Collaboration with healthcare providers, support from loved ones, and personal commitment are key to successful long-term hypertension management.

15.2 Coping with Diagnosis and Treatment

Receiving a diagnosis of hypertension can be overwhelming, and navigating treatment options may add to the stress. However, with the right coping strategies and support, you can manage your condition effectively and maintain a positive outlook. Here's how to cope with the diagnosis and treatment of hypertension.

Understanding Your Condition:

- Take time to learn about hypertension, including its causes, risks, and treatment options. Knowledge is empowering and can alleviate fears or misconceptions.

Develop a Management Plan:

- Work closely with your healthcare provider to develop a comprehensive management plan tailored to your specific needs, preferences, and health goals.

Embrace Lifestyle Changes:

- View lifestyle modifications not as restrictions but as opportunities for enhancing your overall health. Small, incremental changes can lead to significant improvements in blood pressure and well-being.

Medication Adherence:

- Understand the role of each medication prescribed, including how and when to take them, as well as potential side effects. Setting reminders or using a pill organizer can help maintain consistency.

Seek Support:

- Connect with friends, family, or support groups who understand what you're going through. Sharing experiences and receiving encouragement can make managing your condition less daunting.

Stay Active and Engaged:

- Continue engaging in activities you enjoy and explore new hobbies that can help reduce stress and improve your quality of life.

Prioritize Mental Health:

- Recognize that feelings of anxiety or depression are common after a diagnosis. Seeking support from a mental health professional can provide strategies for coping with these emotions.

Communicate Openly:

- Keep open lines of communication with your healthcare team. Don't hesitate to ask questions, express concerns, or discuss any difficulties you're experiencing with your treatment plan.

Monitor Your Progress:

- Regularly monitor your blood pressure at home to track the effectiveness of your management plan. Share these readings with your healthcare provider to make informed adjustments to your treatment.

Adjust Expectations:

- Understand that managing hypertension is a long-term commitment and that fluctuations in blood pressure are normal. Celebrate small victories and be patient with yourself as you make lifestyle adjustments.

Stay Positive:

- Focus on the aspects of your health that you can control and maintain a positive outlook. Remember, hypertension is a manageable condition, and many people live full, active lives with proper care.

Conclusion:

Coping with a diagnosis of hypertension involves education, open communication, support, and a proactive approach to treatment and lifestyle changes. By taking an active role in your health care, seeking support, and focusing on what you can control, you can effectively manage hypertension and lead a healthy life.

15.3 Success Stories and Inspirational Journeys

Hearing about others who have successfully managed their hypertension can be incredibly motivating and reassuring. Success stories provide tangible examples of how adopting healthy lifestyle changes, adhering to treatment plans, and maintaining a positive attitude can lead to significant improvements in blood pressure and overall health. These inspirational journeys highlight the power of perseverance, education, and support in overcoming the challenges associated with hypertension.

John's Story: Embracing Lifestyle Changes

John was diagnosed with hypertension in his early 40s. Initially overwhelmed, he committed to a comprehensive lifestyle overhaul. He started by modifying his diet to include more fruits, vegetables, and whole grains while cutting back on sodium and processed foods. He also began walking every day, gradually increasing his activity level. Over several months, John lost 20 pounds, and his blood pressure readings significantly improved. He credits his success to small, manageable changes and the support of his family.

Maria's Journey: Medication and Mindfulness

Maria struggled with high blood pressure despite being on medication. Realizing that stress was a major contributing factor, she decided to incorporate mindfulness meditation into her daily routine. She also worked with her doctor to adjust her medication. Over time, Maria noticed a decrease in her blood pressure and felt more at peace. She found that mindfulness helped her manage stress more effectively, complementing her medication and contributing to her overall well-being.

Alex's Transformation: From Diagnosis to Marathon Runner

After a hypertension diagnosis, Alex, who had been sedentary for years, decided to make a drastic change. He started with short walks, gradually building up to running. Along the way, he educated himself about heart-healthy nutrition, making significant dietary changes. Two years later, Alex ran his first marathon. His blood pressure had returned to normal levels without medication, a testament to the impact of physical activity and dietary changes.

Linda's Approach: Community Support

Linda found strength in numbers after her diagnosis by joining a local support group for individuals with hypertension. Sharing experiences, tips, and challenges with the group provided her with valuable insights and motivation. She also participated in group exercise sessions, which made staying active more enjoyable. Linda attributes her success in managing her hypertension to the accountability and encouragement she received from her support network.

Conclusion:

These success stories illustrate that while hypertension can be a challenging condition to manage, it is possible to achieve significant improvements through determination, lifestyle modifications, medication adherence, and the power of support. Each journey is unique, but the common thread is the commitment to making positive changes and the resilience to stick with them. Let these stories inspire you to take charge of your health and write your own success story in managing hypertension.

15.4 Exercise: 10 MCQs with Answers at the End

Test your understanding of living with hypertension through these multiple-choice questions. Review the answers at the end for self-assessment.

1. **Long-term management of hypertension primarily involves:**

   A. Temporary medication use

   B. Lifestyle modifications and consistent medication adherence

   C. Surgery as a first-line treatment

   D. Ignoring dietary sodium intake

2. **One effective strategy for coping with a hypertension diagnosis is to:**

   A. Avoid learning about the condition

   B. Work closely with healthcare providers to develop a management plan

C. Isolate from friends and family

D. Increase consumption of processed foods

3. **A success story in managing hypertension often includes:**

A. Giving up after the first setback

B. Significant lifestyle changes and a positive attitude

C. Sole reliance on medication without lifestyle adjustments

D. Refusal to monitor blood pressure at home

4. **Community support for those with hypertension can provide:**

A. Misleading medical advice

B. Emotional support and shared experiences

C. An excuse for non-adherence to treatment plans

D. A platform for commercial product promotion

5. **When building healthy habits to prevent or manage hypertension, it's important to:**

A. Expect immediate results

B. Start with small, manageable changes

C. Only focus on physical activity, ignoring diet

D. Skip regular health check-ups

6. Medication adherence in hypertension management means:

A. Taking medication only when blood pressure is high

B. Consistently taking prescribed medication as directed

C. Using medication as the sole management strategy

D. Avoiding medication to focus on lifestyle changes only

7. The DASH diet is specifically designed to:

A. Increase body weight

B. Lower blood pressure

C. Enhance athletic performance

D. Reduce environmental impact

8. Mindfulness and stress reduction techniques can help manage hypertension by:

A. Increasing stress hormone levels

B. Decreasing stress hormone levels and promoting relaxation

C. Directly lowering cholesterol

D. Raising blood pressure temporarily for stress adaptation

9. A key component of long-term hypertension management is:

A. Ignoring lifestyle and dietary factors

B. Regular monitoring and healthcare appointments

C. Focusing solely on herbal supplements

D. Avoiding physical activity

10. **The role of personalized medicine in hypertension includes:**

A. Using a one-size-fits-all treatment approach

B. Tailoring treatment based on genetic makeup and lifestyle factors

C. Discouraging the use of modern medication

D. Recommending the same diet for all patients

Answers:

1. **B. Lifestyle modifications and consistent medication adherence**

2. **B. Work closely with healthcare providers to develop a management plan**

3. **B. Significant lifestyle changes and a positive attitude**

4. **B. Emotional support and shared experiences**

5. **B. Start with small, manageable changes**

6. **B. Consistently taking prescribed medication as directed**

7. **B. Lower blood pressure**

8. **B. Decreasing stress hormone levels and promoting relaxation**

9. **B. Regular monitoring and healthcare appointments**

10. **B. Tailoring treatment based on genetic makeup and lifestyle factors**

Conclusion

As we've explored the comprehensive journey through understanding, managing, and living with hypertension, it's clear that this condition requires a multifaceted approach. From initial diagnosis to long-term management, each chapter has underscored the importance of medication adherence, lifestyle modifications, support networks, and the evolving landscape of treatments and technologies. The central themes of education, empowerment, and proactive healthcare engagement resonate throughout, offering a blueprint for individuals to navigate the challenges of hypertension effectively.

The journey doesn't end here. The field of hypertension care is continuously advancing, with new research, treatments, and management strategies emerging. Staying informed and engaged with your healthcare team is crucial as you adapt to these changes and optimize your health strategy over time.

Remember, managing hypertension is a collaborative and dynamic process that benefits from a positive outlook, persistence, and adaptability. By leveraging the insights and strategies discussed, you can take meaningful steps towards controlling your blood pressure, reducing the risk of complications, and enhancing your overall quality of life. Embrace the journey with confidence, knowing that each step forward is a step towards better health.

*The best way to thank an author is
to
write a review.*